UNLOCK
your
HEALTH

Live Your Best Life

UNLOCK your HEALTH

Live Your Best Life

MONIQUE JHINGON

authors UPFRONT

*This book is dedicated to my amazing clients
who did the work and proved, again and again,
that optimal health is exquisitely personal,
life-changing, and very much within reach.*

Praise for *Unlock Your Health*

Monique Jhingon artfully walks us through the journey of personalised healthcare through the lens of functional applications. She highlights how we are all bio-individuals and helps to connect us to our unique "why," ultimately enabling us to chart our pathway to better health. Not only is this a great read – Monique is an expert guide who holds our hand as we take the steps to finally feel better.

Andrea Nakayama, Functional Medicine Nutritionist, Founder, CEO Emeritus, Functional Nutrition Alliance

In an age where a mind-boggling and often confusing overload of information on weight loss, exercise, nutrition, and lifestyle is thrown at you from every angle, Monique brings a refreshingly personal approach to optimising your health. No instant gratification, but a measured and holistic approach to being the best version of yourself, health wise. I have seen Monique through years of honing her skills and experience in the field of functional nutrition, and I love that she offers no quick fixes. She is in it for the long haul and her approach is based on solutions that last, by discovering what works for you as an individual. An enduring balance between mind and body, rest and nutrition, lifestyle choices and exercise – *Unlock Your Health* is a valuable tool in uniquely navigating your way to a healthier you.

Anita Shirodkar, Graphic Designer, Author, Entrepreneur

Perfect health and happiness: we all want it! And now this book provides a roadmap to achieving that much-desired state. Monique Jhingon, an experienced functional nutritionist, health writer, and educator, generously shares her personal journey to health and happiness as she explains in simple language, the authoritative science and practical strategies that we can all use to live our lives to the fullest. In the expanding field of body mind science, this book stands out, taking a personalised approach that acknowledges our uniqueness as individuals. No one-size-fits-all solutions here! Informative, inspiring, potentially life-changing, this book is a must read for anyone who wants to optimise their health and get the most out of this "one precious life".

Pip Moran, Artist, Writer, Consultant Editor

MJ simplifies the often complex topic of health and happiness to help create a personalised plan that is own-able and easy to implement. It helped me overcome my sleep challenge and I now wake up each day, rejuvenated and joyful.

Ajay Pahwa, Board Advisor

Monique has accomplished what I miss in many books: it is very personal; we learn a lot about Monique's journey and how her life evolved across the globe. She shares and guides the reader with few words, excellent examples, and a solid step-by-step approach towards self-realisation, helping us to understand what it takes to improve one's overall health and the impact this has on achieving lasting inner happiness. No complicated diet strategies or overly excessive workout regimes are recommended, but rather an approach that is accessible and effective at improving physical and mental balance. *Unlock Your Health* resonated with me because it is written from the bottom of her heart and with lots of her personal self-reflection while encouraging us to follow her guiding example on the road to optimal health and inner contentment.

Ingo Schweder, Founder & CEO GOCO Hospitality, Managing Director Horwath HTL Health & Wellness

Unlock Your Health is easy to digest and high in substance. It offers a 360-degree can-do for creating a whole-self wellness. It removes confusion and adds a personal touch to make its valuable insights relatable and doable for anyone seeking a feel-great lifestyle.

Priscilla Heffelfinger, Co-founder Thrive

CONTENTS

INTRODUCTION

I had just filled a plate with delicious Indian food from the buffet and was making my way back to my table to sit down and eat when a friend approached me. "I am not going to keep you," he said, looking at my plate, "but I just wanted to ask if you could come and meet a friend of mine when you are finished eating. I think he could use your help." We were at a Diwali party hosted by a mutual friend and the atmosphere was festive, food was abundant, and drinks were flowing freely. Which is why I noticed immediately, after arriving at their table a bit later, that the only thing the friend in question had in front of him was a glass of water. I sat down next to him and his wife and we started talking.

Sanjay and his wife were serial expats. He was 46 years old and had been living in Manila for about two years. He told me that the Philippines was the sixth country they had lived in since the start of his career and that they enjoyed their life here. He was a senior executive in a large international company and had a great but demanding job, with long hours and considerable stress.

He was no stranger to the demands of a high-profile job and seemed quite health conscious. He told me he made it a point to balance out his work life with plenty of exercise and time for his family but that, for reasons he didn't understand, he had started struggling with his digestion in the past six months. "I am down to just a handful of homecooked foods these days," he said. "Those few foods are all I can eat without feeling bloated, nauseous, and uncomfortably full. Eating outside of home, and especially from a buffet, is asking for trouble, so I avoid it altogether."

Sanjay had gone to see a doctor, had tests done, and was given medication for his symptoms but none of it had really helped. "I am managing," he said, "but this is not sustainable. I need to turn things around quickly or it's going to impact my life and my work even more and I can't afford for that to happen." After telling him a bit about my work as a functional health and nutrition practitioner and my process for resolving health issues like his, he was more than happy to start working with me.

And so, we started on a personalised health building journey, initially just focusing on nutrition and lifestyle, and implementing changes tailormade to his needs step by step. We streamlined his diet and made sure he was eating plenty of nutrient dense, anti-inflammatory foods that were not causing him symptoms, while at the same time including special supplements and other strategies to restore his digestive function. In as little as two weeks, he happily reported that the bloating and nausea had drastically improved and that he was feeling lighter.

As time progressed Sanjay lost weight, his energy levels increased, and he was feeling a lot less distracted by what was going on with his digestion. By learning what his body most needed and giving it exactly that he transformed his health, which in turn had an enormous direct impact on his confidence, energy, productivity, and focus, and indirectly on the things that mattered most to him: a fulfilling personal life and successful career.

A few months after finishing our work together I bumped into Sanjay at another get-together. This time he was enjoying the food and drinks that were being served. "I feel great and I have some amazing news to share: I was just offered a dream job in Tokyo," he said, beaming. "I am wrapping up work here and my wife and I can't wait for our next adventure. I can't thank you enough for helping me put my health back on track. It has, in more ways than one, transformed my life."

That our health is important, and that optimising your health is a powerful way to improve your quality of life are well known facts. I could share many more stories of clients just like Sanjay. Clients who, as an indirect result of feeling mentally more balanced, losing weight, boosting their energy levels, and thinking more clearly, went on to find new career opportunities, rekindled their marriage, their libido, who finally took that decision to quit their job and start their own business, go on a sabbatical, or set new personal physical performance records.

The benefits of a well-functioning body and mind are endless. But you already knew that. I didn't share Sanjay's story or write this book to convince you to start looking after your health. My guess is that you already are or that you are trying to. I am also not going to tell you exactly what to do to optimise your health. This is not another "diet" book or one-fit-for-all solution. If there is one thing that I have learnt from all my years of working with clients, it is that there is no single magic pill. I know nothing about you, your history, what got you to this point, where you live and have lived, your family history, your health concerns, symptoms, underlying imbalances, genetics, or your environment. There is absolutely no way that I can tell you what to eat and how to live without all that information. And anyone who tries to without these details is not doing you justice. What I can and will show you are the steps you can follow to find your unique path to optimal health and that it is well worth undertaking this journey now before you find yourself in Sanjay's shoes or worse.

We all strive to become better versions of ourselves. We all have hopes and dreams and the desire to live a life full of meaning, connection, creativity, and joy. What we tend to forget is that we are inhabiting a structure that can make or break our journey to becoming our best selves. As Sanjay and many others (maybe you too) who have been in similar situations will tell you: It is not easy to work on personal growth when your body is in pain. When your mind is distracted, anxious or depressed. When you spend all night tossing and turning and all day feeling fatigued. When you are heavy, overweight, depressed. When your attention is continuously drawn to the ache, rumble, or bloating in your stomach. When your mental clarity is obscured by medication, or your skin is constantly itching. Believe me, I know. It is hard to feel truly alive when your body is dragging you down and your mind is unable to focus. And, as I will discuss in the next chapter, suboptimal health and the resulting ripple effects are increasingly common and frankly, staring us all in the face as we grow older.

At the foundation of your journey to achieving all you want out of life, whether that is true happiness, success, financial freedom, or fill in the blank, is a necessary first step: to ensure you are truly the healthiest you can be and continue to be. To be free of aches and pains, full of energy and vigour, to have a calm and focused mind, balanced moods, and a strong digestion. Your goal, first and foremost, is to make sure that this vehicle called your body-mind can support you on your journey to true fulfilment and happiness. Now and in the future.

If you are ready to own your potential and squeeze every bit out of this one precious life, let's begin.

PART 1

SETTING THE STAGE

—◆—

CHAPTER 1

A REALITY CHECK

A scary reality

Health problems are rampant. Global health statistics are truly alarming, and what is even more frightening is that these statistics include just the population data for diagnosed health conditions. What is not considered in the already scary statistics are sub-clinical, lingering health issues that doctors can't fit into a well-defined diagnostic box and that people have learnt to live with.

If you had a chance to sit down and spend some time with everyone you encountered, you would soon realise that there are very few people who don't have a health complaint or two. You'll find (as I did) that your hairdresser has chronic eye irritation. A colleague has been told he is on the verge of type 2 diabetes, your successful friend can't get rid of his skin rashes, the receptionist at the doctor's office deals with chronic fatigue, the cashier at the grocery store has chronic recurring UTIs, your boss takes antacids every night, and your cousin struggles with insomnia.

What is even scarier is that many of these low-grade chronic issues are accepted as normal. As long as we are able to function, these health challenges may be annoying, but they are not thought of as being unwell. Even though in reality, any symptom is a sign that there are underlying imbalances in your body and that ignoring or failing to correct these imbalances at the root can eventually result in even greater imbalances and other symptoms.

We have collectively learnt to accept as normal a standard of health that is way below what is possible. We live with aches and pains, with itchy and patchy skins, we ignore a digestive system that sends us signals, like bloating and heartburn. We have learnt to live with mood swings, feeling low, suboptimal sleep, low level fatigue, recurring UTIs. We have forgotten what it is like to truly thrive. It's usually only when the low-level rumble becomes too loud to ignore that we take notice and are driven to act. That action usually begins with a visit to our doctor, maybe a few blood tests to look for answers, sometimes a diagnosis and often a bunch of prescriptions to manage our symptoms. These prescription pills or lotions reduce the severity of our symptoms and on we go with our lives. Until another symptom pops up and we repeat the process.

Recognising the importance of nutrition and lifestyle factors, we also may embark on a journey to find the right diet, supplement, or other natural interventions that help us manage or resolve our nagging health challenges.

Only to end up feeling very confused with the often widely conflicting and opposing theories about the right diet approach, food eliminations, detoxes, and other interventions.

A quick Google search on a particular health issue or health goal will throw up plenty of quick tips and diet solutions that promise to cure you of your ailment. Proponents of specific diets or techniques very convincingly tell you that theirs is the best approach. These people have found their magic formula and assume that it is the same formula that will help everyone feel better or lose weight. Their enthusiasm is infectious, and it undoubtedly comes from the right place. They (or at least most of them) are driven by a desire to help the world experience what they experienced. A very noble act – only in reality, it doesn't work. Everyone is unique and as such needs a unique approach. I will get into the how of this in more detail later. In the meantime, let's have a look at some of the reasons why we are, collectively, dealing with suboptimal health and/or a failure to thrive.

An evolutionary mismatch

We humans have taken a long time to get to where we are now. Millions of years, in fact. The majority of which we lived in ways that are very different from how we are living today. Our ancestors lived with the cycles of nature and the seasons, they were at one with their environment and lived off the earth – by hunting for wild animals, catching wild fish and gathering whatever plant foods were available at any point in time. They woke up with the dawn and went to sleep when the sun set. They lived in clean environments, free from any of the pollutants that we are dealing with today.

From an evolutionary perspective it has been a relatively short period of time where our way of living changed quite drastically. Roughly about 10,000 years ago agriculture began, and we started relying on different types of foods and lifestyles. Further changes happened with the birth of technology and if we look at our lives now compared to the lives of our ancestors, it looks drastically different. But while our circumstances changed, our genes did not. We are biochemically and structurally the same species that thrived in natural surroundings for millions of years, yet we are now living under circumstances that our bodies are technically not designed for. We are, to put it bluntly, genetic misfits.

We are disconnected from nature, much less exposed to natural sunlight, and we sleep in airconditioned rooms. We sit a lot: when we commute to work, at work, when at home. We are dealing with chronic stress, we eat foods that are flown to us from all corners of the world, regardless of the season. Those same foods have been genetically modified, sprayed with pesticides, and packed in plastic. Our groceries stores are full of heavily processed packaged foods that contain unnatural ingredients.

Don't get me wrong, our modern world offers great

things that we should be very thankful for. Moving to a deserted corner of the world and recreating our ancestral way of living is not the answer and I don't believe we need to reverse what we have achieved. We can and should make use of modern comforts.

What we do need is awareness of the fact that we are genetically mismatched with our current circumstances. While technology and science advanced rapidly, our genes stayed the same and that is a big reason we are experiencing a health crisis. What we need most is to learn ways to manage this disconnect. Awareness is the first step. From there you can start to find ways to overcome the obstacles you are faced with.

A pill for every ill

Some of the most brilliant achievements we have made in the past few decades have been in the area of medicine and healthcare. It is mind-blowing to think about the abilities we have today to replace organs, repair injuries, perform an open heart or brain surgery, treat cancer, and find effective vaccines for viruses virtually overnight. We are so fortunate to have access to medical care the way we know it.

Where we have fallen behind is in the management and prevention of chronic health conditions. We have so-called solutions to common problems in the form of pharmaceutical drugs, but these typically only treat the symptoms. And as I mentioned earlier, where there are symptoms – from high cholesterol levels, weight gain, aches and pains, skin conditions, inflammation, fatigue, to bloating and acid reflux, there are underlying imbalances that drive these symptoms.

A pill for every ill – the way modern medicine approaches our health issues, is hardly a successful way to resolve these root cause imbalances. And neither is the endless journey from specialist to specialist, who look at a part of the problem without recognising that everything in the body is connected.

I learnt all this the hard way.

My story

I was born and brought up in a small town in the Netherlands. I had a wonderful, happy, and stable childhood. The town I grew up in was small enough to bike everywhere: to the grocery store, school, a friend's house, the swimming pool in summer, or horse-riding class. On the right end of our street began a stretch of farmland and the forest and natural lakes were nearby.

I was a quiet, introverted child. An avid reader who liked to disappear in books or the outdoors. Some of my fondest childhood memories include growing plants on the windowsill of my bedroom, drying and identifying wild flowers, lying outside on a blanket in our garden on warm summer days and watching the plants and flowers around me move gently in the breeze while bees and butterflies buzzed around frantically. Or going on foraging trips to the forest with my mom to pluck wild blackberries, which she would use to make fresh jam.

My parents both helped cultivate that love of the outdoors; Sunday walks in the nearby forests or winter ice skating on the frozen lakes were a part of life. Summer holidays were spent camping and hiking in the mountains of Switzerland or Austria. Additionally, my mom helped instil an appreciation for music, healthy food, and cooking. She also brought spirituality, yoga, and self-awareness into my life at an early age. Yoga, meditation, and eastern philosophy had made their inroads into the western world. Writers such as Wayne Dyer were hugely popular, and my mother explored and shared many of her experiences with me. When I was in high school, I would come home and use her yoga books to practice headstands and other poses in the living room and when she was given a meditation mantra at one of the workshops she attended I borrowed her mantra and practiced meditation in my bedroom. Books such as *I'm OK – You're OK* taught me about taking charge of your inner life and opened me up to the science of self-actualisation.

And then I became a teenager and suddenly none of that was important anymore. What became important were friends, boyfriends, clothes, make-up, parties. Throughout high school and while in college that part of life took over even if in the background the pull and fascination with the inner world lingered on.

It was during my Masters in France that I met my

now husband and ended up taking the life-changing decision to follow him to India, his country of birth, to get married and start a life together. It was one of the best and at the same time one of the most difficult things I have done. The differences between the life I knew and the life I moved into were so huge that, especially in the first year, I spent many nights wondering how I was ever going to fit in. Never did I regret my decision and I absolutely loved learning all about India's rich culture, foods, places, meeting new people. My husband is the opposite of me in many ways: he is outgoing, loves the limelight, and thrives on being with people. His family and friends welcomed me with open arms and made me feel at home from the first moment. I missed my parents deeply and trips home were quite expensive and therefore, limited, as we were building a life for ourselves, but my husband showered me with love and care and introduced me to people who I still count among my closest friends.

Shortly after our marriage I started working with a large international bank in Mumbai. I travelled across the country as part of my role in Customer Quality Service Management and learnt about the vast differences that exist between cultures and cuisines within the same country and the amazing hospitality of the Indian people. I loved Indian food and happily tried whatever was offered to me, sometimes to my own detriment: bouts of stomach infection, some worse than others, were a regular affair.

It didn't stop me from enjoying food; eating with friends was an important part of our lives and I learnt how to navigate spice like a pro.

I spent a total of seven and a half years in India before we moved to the Maldives, where my husband was given the responsibility of opening a high-end resort on one of the islands. Our eldest son was two years old at the time and I had just found out I was pregnant with our second son. It meant I had to stop working but I was ready to spend more time being a mom. It had been quite challenging to navigate a full-time job with a small child and I was ready for some time off.

The two years that we lived in the Maldives were blissful. Every morning I would wake up and look out onto the jetty that extended into the bluest of oceans and count myself lucky for living in paradise. For two years straight, the boys and I walked around barefoot, with as little clothing as possible. We swam in the ocean every day, played in the sand. I learnt diving and became an advanced open water diver and explored the beautiful life that lies beneath the surface of the ocean. It was in the Maldives that I took my first yoga class. The class was held on a platform in the middle of the ocean and as I bent and stretched my body to the sounds of the waves splashing, I became one with my breath and I knew I had come home.

It was also in the Maldives that a friend, Ashfer, the executive chef in the resort, lent me a book on Ayurveda and it opened me up to the world of natural healing and looking at my body in a whole different light: a unique combination of energy and forces that interact with one another and are influenced by our environment. I was dealing with lingering digestive issues and a few other minor health complaints at the time and knew instinctively that the answers lay deeper. Maybe Ayurveda was the key to figuring it all out.

We left the Maldives after two wonderful years with a bag full of experiences and for me, a newfound love of yoga. Singapore was our next stop. After taking time to settle in, setting up our new home and getting the boys used to their new school and environment, I contemplated going back to work but decided I wanted to be there for my children. While I was clear about that decision, there was an underlying yearning to discover my purpose in life. After some soul searching, I decided that my true purpose in that moment was to be the best mom and partner I could be, and I made peace with that.

At the same time, I started to pursue the things I was drawn to. I did a yoga teacher training course and studied with a spiritual teacher. In addition, I started a search for answers to my chronic digestive issues that had slowly been getting worse. I now frequently doubled over with stomach pain. It was no longer just my digestion that was troubling me: I had skin rashes, acne, I had difficulties falling asleep at night, I was moody and had a tough time getting out of bed in the morning. I had come to the point that I described earlier: the low-level rumble had become too loud to ignore and I kicked off my search through conventional medicine.

My first stop: a general practitioner. He looked at my skin, took note of my digestive complaints and prescribed a cream. Before leaving I asked him why he thought I had these problems. He thought for a moment and proceeded to tell me it could be anything, maybe even the hot and humid climate here in Singapore. I left the clinic none the wiser and a tad bit more frustrated.

Next stop: a gastroenterologist who performed a colonoscopy, which came back all clear. He told me everything was in order and sent me home without any real advice.

Third stop: a dermatologist. I walked away from the clinic with another ointment for my skin rashes and that was that.

Fourth stop: a gynaecologist who was lovely and a bit more thorough. She ran a hormone panel and sat down with me to explain what was going on with my hormones: I was oestrogen dominant. She talked a bit about the implications of hormonal imbalances, about possible contributing factors, diet, and lifestyle factors and prescribed a bio-identical progesterone cream.

In the meantime, during this entire process of searching for answers (and not really finding any) I became obsessed with food. I believed that it played a role in what was going on with me and I started reading every diet book I could get my hands on. I tried to eat according to my Ayurvedic constitution, then experimented with the blood type diet. When that didn't quite do the trick, I embarked on a vegan, raw diet and turned my kitchen into a juicing, de-hydrating, sprouting lab. While it felt great to be eating clean, my digestion became explosively worse. I refused to admit it was the diet, thinking I was taking my system through a much-needed detox and that this was how it was supposed to be. I applauded every bout of diarrhoea, thinking it was my body's way of getting rid of toxins.

Somewhere during that time, my husband and I decided we needed a break. He had been tasked with the temporary closure and renovation of one of the leading 5-star hotels in the country, and it had been busy and stressful. I had been taking care of the kids while dealing with my health issues and so we decided to run off for a long weekend to Bali. My in-laws had planned a visit and we coordinated it so that they could look after the boys while we spent a few days on a romantic get-away.

The hotel we stayed in was gorgeous. We were in a luxurious villa in the lush tropical gardens of the property, and everything was perfect. The morning of our first day there, we woke up, went for breakfast, and then returned to our rooms to plan the rest of the day. I had woken up with a slight headache and my stomach was hurting, so I lay down as my husband was going through the options and without realising, I fell back asleep. I woke up three hours later, my husband patiently waiting for me in the garden with a cup of coffee, and despite that nap, I still felt completely depleted of all energy. I had absolutely no desire to do anything except lay in bed and that is how I spent most of our romantic weekend: with a pain in my head and my stomach hurting, fatigued and depressed about the state I was in.

Somewhere during that weekend, I realised this could not go on. I was tired, frustrated, and scared: what was going on with me? Was it something serious? Like cancer? Why was no one able to give me answers? Why wasn't anything I tried working? I realised I had to figure this out on my own. Conventional medicine was clearly not able to give me any real answers and whatever diet approaches that were out there were not working for me either. My health issues had started to significantly impact the quality of my life and the people around me. I made a commitment to myself to do everything necessary to find the answers and restore my health, energy, and vitality. I owed it to my husband, my children, and myself.

What will it take?

Perhaps my story resonates. You may be or have been in a similar situation, dealing with nagging health issues and reaching a roadblock with the available options. Like me, you may be confused with all the conflicting advice that is out there and you sense that what you need is an approach that is unique to your situation. The fact that you are reading this book means you are intrigued and interested in restoring or further optimising your health and your life. It means you recognise that there is a better way, and you are hungry to know what that way may be for you.

I spent many years finding a solution to my problems and then several more years turning that process into a roadmap for others. I have worked with countless people, helping them find their personal way to better health, and I have realised there are two kinds of people: those that, like me, have decided "this can't go on". They have a wake-up call or experience a strong call to action, the way I did in Bali. If this is you, you are ready to do what it takes to find answers and learn how to thrive and squeeze everything you can out of life. This wake-up call can come in many forms. For me, it was the realisation that I was not able to fully live my life, that I was being held back. For others it can be witnessing disease or a health scare in their circle of friends or family, which reminds them of their own mortality.

And then there is yet another set of people who have an innate drive to spend this one and precious life of theirs in the most optimal way; they have things to do, goals to achieve and they know they need this vehicle called the body to be in tip top condition to support them through their life's journey.

Which category do you fit in to? What will it take for

you to go on this journey, get to truly know yourself and learn how to thrive in a world that is no longer conducive to thriving? Because the journey to self-optimisation is not for the fainthearted and in the next chapter I will explain why.

CHAPTER 2

KNOW WHAT YOU'RE UP AGAINST

Not for the fainthearted

Before embarking on a journey, you want to familiarise yourself with the landscape and you want to be prepared for roadblocks, challenges, hurdles – anything that can either be avoided by being prepared properly or that can be navigated with the help of some tools that you bring along in your backpack.

The journey of a health seeker or self-optimiser is not for the fainthearted. It is ridden with obstacles, some of which stem from within but most of which are a result of the society that we live in. It is important that you walk into this with eyes wide open and an ability to recognise the forces that are against you.

Information overload

Let's start with hurdle number one: the information overload. When I started my journey to find answers to my challenges, I quickly began to realise that there is a lot of information out there. And while it can be a wonderful thing to read, explore, and educate yourself, it can quickly result in utter confusion and overwhelm, as I hinted at in the previous chapter. Why is it that there are countless people who have found their solution in eating a vegan diet while there are others who are miraculously cured from their symptoms when they eat a carnivorous diet? When you dive into the logic behind all these often very opposing dietary strategies, theoretically they all make sense. You can find truth in the logic of all these different approaches and most of them have evidence to back up their claims. And broad dietary strategies like vegan, paleo, keto, or the Mediterranean diet are only the beginning – scan the internet and you will find endless permutations and combinations, all of which sound plausible and very convincing. You can do quizzes to identify your "type" – from blood type to body type or metabolic type – and find various ways to put yourself into a particular category that then will provide you with your ideal diet.

When you delve deeper into nutrition science and look at the many research studies that are conducted over the years, the confusion continues. Taking weight loss as an example: studies have shown a favourable outcome on weight loss by adopting a low-fat diet and at the same time, other studies show that eating a high fat, low carb diet promotes weight loss. How can you possibly make sense of this all?

Even when I work with clients who wholeheartedly

decide to take on a personalised approach in working with me and completely buy into the strategy that has been crafted exclusively for them, I still receive the occasional message asking what I think about "metabolic typing" or the vegan approach. It is understandable: when you hear someone's success story in restoring their health, losing weight, or running a marathon, your mind starts questioning whether this is not something you should be trying.

In other words: the first hurdle you want to prepare for is the information overload hurdle. And the best way to do that is to approach everything with curiosity and openness but to stay committed to what you have set out to do: finding **your** unique and personalised approach to eating and living – the "diet" and lifestyle that is appropriate for you according to your current health status, your genetic code, your life history, your environment, and your goals.

Everyone knows better

The second hurdle comes in the form of people around you that have advice, judgments, and insecurities. What you must do is build up a harness to protect yourself from these well-meaning individuals.

There are a few different categories of people: those that come with loving advice and tips. These are the people that have found their unique approach and truly believe this is the answer for everyone. They mean well and you can hear them out, thank them for their advice and then move on. Another set of people will unconsciously try to sabotage your efforts. This fun loving, social bunch will want you to have a drink at their cocktail party or share their dessert at dinner. They can't understand why you choose to say no and consider it boring when you don't participate in the fun.

One of my clients, an entrepreneurial start-up consultant, struggled with this. While entertaining his clients, wine would flow freely, and he admitted that alcohol helped to loosen the mood. At such dinners deals are made, mergers and acquisitions are initiated, and alcohol helps to loosen up the vibe, and doing business becomes easier. Saying no at this point felt to him like he was obstructing the process. Other clients have walked into a dinner party determined to avoid drinking, only to be persuaded by the host after repeatedly being told to "come on, just have one!"

People may feel judged by the choices you make. Perhaps they instinctively know that they should not be ordering dessert or eating a bag of chips and they perceive your refusal to partake in these extravaganzas as a silent attack on their habits.

Junk food is everywhere

And finally, let's not forget the larger forces that are upon us – the food companies that have created products meant to create food addictions and that use heavy advertising to feed on those addictions. Think of fast-food restaurants at every corner, supermarkets that put chocolate bars near the checkout counters, and the lack of healthy options when dining out as some of the pitfalls you are working against.

To summarise, when you are deciding to do what it takes to be your optimal best, you will feel like an exception to the norm. You are a trailblazer, a rebel, a deviant. And society does not conform to the exceptions, so you will, therefore, have to walk your path with strength and conviction and yes, tools that will help you stay the course. When I take you through the 6-step process I will provide you with these tools and all the other things you need to be successful.

Muddy waters

You may have heard of the Blue Zones. These are areas in the world that have a higher than usual number of healthy and long-living people. From Okinawa in Japan to Icaria in Greece, the Blue Zones are spread across the world, but they share certain characteristics that have been the focus of researchers determined to find the recipe to health and longevity.

There are many lessons to be learnt from the people living in these Blue Zones; lessons we can incorporate in our lives to be healthier and live longer. But there is an important distinction between us (you and me and most of the people we know) and these Blue Zone centenarians. They were born, brought up in their Blue Zone areas, and stayed there, living simple lives, with access to the same fresh and seasonal foods, lifestyles that naturally included plenty of outdoor movement, clean air, and a stable community of relatives and friends.

On the contrary, chances are you are not living in the same place you were born. Your diet probably includes some of the foods you grew up with but also plenty of international cuisines, ranging from sushi to Indian food to Chinese. Most of your physical movement happens in the gym, a few times a week. The rest of the time you are quite sedentary, working indoors, at a desk, behind a computer. You are probably living in a big city, surrounded by high rise buildings, roads, and traffic. The air you breathe is not clean mountain air but polluted city air. And that is not the only source of toxins: the produce you buy is sprayed with pesticides, your work and home environment are full of harmful chemicals. The grocery store where you buy your food has produce from all over the world, all year round.

When I take a quick glance through the list of clients that I have worked with over the years, there is not even one that doesn't fit this bill. They are all expats that, like me, have taken their genetic code across the world into different climates, cultures, foods. I have worked with senior executives who were born and brought up in Northern Europe and are now living in Singapore, Manila, or Colombo. Indians who have moved around the world, living in a different city every couple of years, from Tokyo to Hong Kong and Dubai. I myself have lived in 8 different countries over the past 25 years. And it is hard for all of us to imagine a world without global cuisines, travel, boardrooms, commutes, and the stress that comes with all of it.

In other words, things are muddled up and that makes it so much harder to figure out what your body needs to thrive. Unlike the centenarians that live in their Blue Zones, you must navigate the complexity of modern, global living and the toxic soup that is your environment.

It makes sense to take a moment and realise the magnitude of this. The answer is not to pack your bags and go back home. You would not want your life to be any different. It is amazing and wonderful that we can experience global lives and that we have access to technology. But it is important to realise what you're up against and how all of this can impact your ability to truly know yourself and what you need to thrive.

The missing pieces

Self-knowledge is power. It is, as I will explain in more detail later, the key to finding your unique recipe for becoming your healthiest, best self. Going back to my Blue Zone example, the people that live in these areas don't have to embark on a self-discovery journey to find out what their bodies need. They are in touch with their roots, their environment, their community, the earth that they live on. Their routine, their eating habits, the food that is available to them has been the same all their lives. They have a certain time in the day for work, time to socialise, time to contribute to the community, time to eat, sleep. Much less technology to navigate, times zones to bridge, or social media accounts to manage.

Our lives are a whole lot more complicated. Work-life balance is often missing, many of us are cut off from the natural environment we live in. We spend our time indoors, in climate-controlled environments or inside cars or other modes of transportation. We barely see natural sunlight unless we try, and we have many of our social interactions via a screen. We are on the go from the time we get up, moving from one task to another, and we spend much of our free time watching what everyone else is doing via social media. As you will see, connecting is crucial to the process of self-optimisation: connecting to the environment you live in, the cycles of nature, people in your community, and most importantly, connecting to yourself.

Catherine, my client, was professionally very successful. Her career in education had taken her across the world, and she was proud of what she had achieved. But it had come at a cost. When we first spoke, Catherine was heavily overweight, she had just recovered from knee surgery, and she was dealing with all kinds of health issues. "I have spent my entire adult life looking after others," she told me. "My family, my employees, my students and their parents, and in the process, I have neglected myself. I have no idea how I let it get to this point but I do know that I feel disconnected to this body and I need to re-connect and start taking care of it."

We discussed what had stopped her from taking care of herself and the list included lack of time, lack of clarity about what to do to, and, she admitted, also a lack of self-love. These missing pieces I see in many of my clients: lack of time and lack of clarity are obvious, but a lack of self-love is not usually identified as a blocking factor to being your optimal self.

If you truly love and value yourself, you value your own happiness and wellbeing, you take care of you own needs, you set healthy boundaries, and you put your physical and emotional wellbeing first. Time and clarity are relatively easy roadblocks to tackle. Self-love: not always so straightforward. This self-sabotaging feeling of "I am not enough" is often ingrained in us from childhood and it is a conscious or subconscious belief that is keeping us from truly living our most optimal lives.

To summarise, certain challenges can and will present themselves on your journey. Being aware of them is going to help you recognise them for what they are when they arise. All these challenges can be overcome if you have the right strategies in place and the right tools in your backpack, and I will share with you everything that I have successfully used in my own life and with my clients.

—◆—

CHAPTER 3

A BETTER WAY

The power of personalisation

Now that you have a vision for yourself, and an awareness of the challenges you are faced with in our modern world and our current approach to healthcare, it is time to look at a better way to approach self-optimisation. A way that recognises that the world around us is ever changing and not always to our benefit. That we are all uniquely positioned within this world, both genetically and because of our life stories. That modern science is beginning to recognise our bio-individuality and that we can make use of the research and the exciting new tools that are rapidly emerging to help create a truly personalised approach.

In 2017 a ground-breaking research study was published in the journal *Cell*. The study had taken place over a period of two years with 800 participants, with the aim to identify the benefits of a personalised approach to nutrition. Participants were first analysed on many markers, ranging from blood test results to their genetics to the composition of their gut microbiome, which are the trillions of micro-organisms that live in our digestive tract and that play a big role in many of our biological processes. They were then tracked to identify individualised blood sugar responses to food. Chronically elevated blood sugar levels are a risk factor for diseases such as type 2 diabetes and are also linked to metabolic issues such as obesity, hypertension, non-alcoholic fatty liver disease, elevated triglycerides, and cardiovascular disease. Diet heavily influences blood glucose levels, and it is well understood that a diet that keeps blood sugar levels balanced is important for health.

All this information was analysed with the use of machine learning models that helped to generate algorithms capable of predicting a person's blood sugar response to different food based on factors such as their genetic profile, lifestyle factors, body composition, and gut microbiome composition. The researchers had picked weight loss as the end goal for personalised nutrition interventions, which is correlated to blood sugar control.

The results of the study showed a few very important things: first, that each individual person had unique responses to different foods. For example, one person's blood sugar level would spike after eating potatoes but not rice, another person would respond more strongly to tomatoes and not potatoes. The second important finding was that a person's unique mix of personal features and microbiome composition could help predict that person's blood glucose response and therefore their "ideal" diet for blood sugar control and weight management.

For the first time in history a scientific research study proved that there is no one perfect diet for humans, but that the perfect diet is unique for every single person. And it showed that we are well on our way to create the technology to help us figure this out.

N=1

When research studies are conducted it is always with a number of subjects. That number is represented with the letter n. In the study mentioned above, n=800. Typically, the larger the number of participants, the better the study as you have more data to draw conclusions. In personalised nutrition, it has become clear that the best study is that of n=1: you are the subject of your own study. There is no doctor, dietician, friend, or book that can tell you exactly what you need to feel optimal. Your optimal diet is unique to you, and it is dependent on your genetic code, your current imbalances, your life story, your cultural background, the environment that you live in, your state of health, your age, your movement, sleep, and the list goes on.

It is intriguing to think that one day we will have easy access to the kind of technology used in a study like the one described above. However, it will take a while before we get to the point where a computer or app can tell us what to eat. And there is obviously more to the story:

it isn't just food that influences our health. Our ever-changing environment also influences how we feel and our propensity for disease. And so do our stress levels, our sleep patterns, our exercise and movement patterns, our relationships, sense of purpose, and spiritual connection. The personalised diet study is an important step to help us understand the need for personalisation and it provides scientific proof that we hold the answers inside us. Not in popular diet trends or books or people that tell us what to eat or how to live. And it points at some very important factors that can help us determine how to go about finding our unique approach to optimal health, even at this point and without having access to artificial intelligence.

The foundation for a personalised approach

When I returned from my trip to Bali, where I had my "call to action", I embarked on a long search for answers to my chronic health issues. I continued to experiment with nutrition and alternative healing therapies, and while some of it helped a bit, I didn't quite manage to fully resolve my issues.

It was not long after that I walked into the clinic of a naturopath in Singapore, who took one look at me, reviewed my health history and my symptoms, and told me I had a leaky gut. Leaky gut, or the more accurate medical term "hyper intestinal permeability", is now a common and well-recognised condition but at the time it wasn't. I had never heard of it and I soon found out that conventional medicine didn't even consider it to be a real "thing".

My naturopath explained it to me: the lining of our digestive tract is made up of a thin layer of cells that are tightly packed together. This barrier essentially separates the outside world from the inside of our bodies. What is let in through the barrier is tightly controlled by internal mechanisms. When the gut is hyper permeable, these cells are no longer tightly packed together; spaces have been formed between the cells through which molecules that are not supposed to can pass into our blood stream, which triggers our immune system.

He confirmed his diagnosis by doing a test via a lab in Australia and told me to stop eating gluten, a component of wheat. He gave me a list of foods to avoid, and that list included foods such as pasta, cake, cookies, bread. I remember looking at him in disbelief: BREAD was the issue? I was Dutch! I had grown up on bread. Surely, if bread wasn't right for me, I would have noticed earlier?

Despite my disbelief, I went along with his advice and soon began to experience relief from some of my symptoms. My digestion calmed down and my skin began to clear up and I noticed an overall improvement in my energy. This doctor had managed to uncover one of my root causes and I had slowly started to heal. In my mind, a question remained: why did my gut decide to go "leaky" suddenly?

My dedicated search and learning continued and over the years that followed I began to put the pieces of the puzzle together. I came to understand that the health issues I had been dealing with resulted from a combination of different things. First, my unique make-up – or my genetics. I had been born into this world with a particular genetic code that contained some variants that made me more susceptible to certain health issues. One of these variants was related to gluten intolerance. I learnt that genes alone don't necessarily decide that these health issues are expressed. That it is the external environment that can trigger the expression of such genes. This is also known as epigenetics. In other words: it was my life story and various environmental influences that had created a perfect storm.

When I looked back at my life history, I realised that there had been several environmental influences that had played a role in the manifestation of my health issues. For starters, I had taken my Northern European body and genetic code across the world into hot and humid surroundings. I had experienced several circumstances that had compromised the balance of my gut microbiome: from frequent courses of antibiotics for recurring ear infections as a child to bouts of gastroenteritis during my first year of living in India that were treated with more antibiotics. It was likely that my gut and the microbes that lived there had never fully recovered from the various assaults.

Later on, when I was studying functional diagnostics and ran a few root cause functional tests on myself, I uncovered lingering bacterial and parasite infections, a severely compromised digestive system that had been unable to break down food properly, nutrient deficiencies and more.

During this entire process I realised I had to stop looking for the right "diet" but rather start using nutritional and other interventions in such a way that I was able to restore my unique root cause imbalances. This approach worked and I started feeling like me again: vibrant, energetic, focused, and happy. I then proceeded to identify a long-term sustainable approach of eating and living that was in line with my genetic make-up, my circumstances, my love of different cuisines, my weak links, and my ever-changing environment.

And that process is what I believe everyone should go through. It is the only way to really get to know yourself, your imbalances, your genetic strengths and weaknesses, to make sense of your life story, and to set yourself up for a lifetime of health and happiness. It is the foundation for your self-optimisation journey. And even if you are not currently struggling with symptoms, you can prevent health issues by engaging in this process now. By learning how to support your unique self and the microbes that reside within your body and by learning to tune in and become more mindful. All of this will help you to catapult yourself into the dream life you have envisioned for yourself. In Chapter 5 you will learn more about the three elements that are an inherent part of this process.

A better healthcare system

The little town I grew up in had only a few of everything. A few hairdressers, two grocery stores, two schools, a butcher, a music store, two dentists, and two doctors. One of those, the one closest to where we lived, was our family doctor.

Dr. van de Water had a clinic adjoining his home, with a small pharmacy managed by his wife. I was friends with his daughter, who was in the same school and class as me. He was a man of very few words but kind and thorough and he practised medicine the way we all know it: he would diagnose the issue and prescribe medicine to help resolve it. If you were dealing with a health issue you would visit the clinic; if the situation was bad enough, he would come pay a visit to your home during his rounds around town.

One of the advantages of being a family doctor in a small town was that he knew all his patients well. He had seen you through your childhood illnesses, ear infections, skin issues, cuts, and bruises. He probably knew about breakups, relationship issues, and financial troubles in families. He treated every member of the family, and he knew the life story of each and every one of his patients, and I am sure he used that information as a valuable tool to prescribe the right intervention or offer a word of advice.

When I left the town I had grown up in to go study in a different part of the Netherlands, and later when I went to live abroad, the experience of dealing with doctors became quite different. I no longer had a family doctor. In India and most of the other countries in Asia you went straight to a specialist. Doctors still diagnosed and prescribed medicine but besides a quick review of your symptoms they knew nothing about you, your life, or your family. The interaction always felt clinical and impersonal, nothing like how it was when I was growing up.

When I experienced my health issues and started seeing one specialist after the other, having 10-minute consultations, receiving prescription medication without any clear answers, I began to realise that something was wrong with the way medicine was practised. It was an approach based on the assumption that the body was made up of individual parts and each specialist focused on their area of expertise. It asked **what** was wrong with you, never digging deeper to understand why. It assumed that symptoms just happen, and that disease just had to be managed with a one size fits all approach.

In my search for answers, I stumbled on a more holistic, functional approach and when I did, it was as if I had finally come home. This way of practising medicine and nutrition recognised that everything in the body is connected, that no symptom is normal but a sign of underlying imbalances. It recognises that everyone is unique and needs to be supported accordingly. It uses natural therapies first and pharmaceutical interventions second, when truly needed. A good functional practitioner takes time to understand your background, your story, your family history, all your current complaints. They ask about your sleep, your stress, your exercise pattern. They connect the dots and look for underlying imbalances. A good functional practitioner will talk to you about diet and lifestyle. They become your partner in your journey to optimal health. They aim to get to know you, just like our small-town family doctor knew his patients.

The rise of Functional Healthcare is real and unstoppable. It is the way of the future for healthcare and prevention. It does not replace conventional medicine; it complements it by being preventative in nature and more effectively dealing with chronic issues versus acute conditions. In a perfect world everyone has access to a functional healthcare practitioner, a partner who keeps an eye on your health, can help you identify the underlying imbalances, and steers you in the right direction with regard to your diet and lifestyle choices.

A glimpse of the future

With the growing recognition of the importance of a functional and personalised healthcare model has come an explosion in tests and tools that support this way of practising healthcare. You can now run tests that show you your genetic strengths and weaknesses. You can order a full analysis of your gut microbiome and see where there are imbalances. You can run tests that show nutrient deficiencies, or toxic burden. You can get a detailed overview of your hormones, mineral levels, digestive function, immune or neurotransmitter imbalances.

It is now possible to get a glimpse inside the "black box" that is your body and understand where and how you need to support yourself. In addition to these functional testing options there is an explosion in devices that help you track various aspects of your health in relatively simple ways. I will go into these in more detail in the second part of this book, where I outline the steps for personalising your self-optimisation approach. But for now, know that there are many tools available to you and it will get even better as we move into a future of personalised healthcare where you are in the driver's seat of your own health, supported by an array of tools, trackers, and a team of allied functional healthcare practitioners.

CHAPTER 4

SHATTERING MYTHS

In my own life, through witnessing others and by working with clients, I have come across some common beliefs that are self-limiting, sometimes outright false, and yet they seem to stick around like gum on your shoes. I am going to take some time to call out these beliefs for what they really are: myths that must be busted to allow you to reach your goals.

Myth 1: Being healthy is boring and restrictive

One of the reasons people ignore nagging signs and symptoms or choose pharmaceutical interventions over diet and lifestyle changes is that they fear having to give up the good things in life. We take immense pleasure in a good meal, a glass of wine, smoking a cigar, and we are terrified that we are going to have to give up these things to pursue long-lasting good health. We fear life is boring without these short-lived pleasures.

Last summer my husband and I met up with close

friends in Florence, Italy for a 5-day trip to celebrate our friends' birthdays. We had a fabulous time, scrolling through the streets, watching Andrea Bocelli perform live in his hometown, dining al fresco, sipping cocktails, having meaningful conversations, eating freshly made pastas, and finishing our meals with a gelato and a nightcap. In other words: we lived it up big time.

I am a firm believer that doing so occasionally is a part of a healthy lifestyle. Life is all about balance. If you have put in place habits that support your health on an on-going basis, you are currently healthy, strong and without issues; if you know your non-negotiables (more on this later) you can be flexible. If, on the other hand, you are (as an example) pre-diabetic, overweight, dealing with chronic allergies and gut issues you need to FIRST restore your underlying imbalances. You are going to have to be careful with your diet and lifestyle choices for a while until balance is restored. Once your health is restored, you are going to have to identify the things that you need to do and the things you need to avoid most of the time to stay at your best. When you are back to feeling healthy, you will have built some resilience to step out of your normal routine and have that glass of wine, or tuck into that birthday cake – you will know what works for you and what doesn't.

When you are feeling strong and energetic, vibrant, and alive, focused and clear, you will want to keep it that way. Your choices will be different because you won't want to jeopardise the way you are feeling. Your taste buds will have changed, you won't like the feeling you have when you wake up the morning after a bender because you have experienced what it feels like and what you are able to accomplish when you wake up fresh and with a zest for life.

Health is so much more than being at an optimal weight or eating a healthy diet, exercising every day. The general definition according to the World Health Organisation is that health is a state of complete mental, physical, and emotional well-being. But rather than defining it in general terms, you will have to decide what it means to you. Does it mean waking up every morning feeling fresh and positive with a zest for life? Or having a healthy glow on your face, wearing a well-cut suit or dress with confidence? Staying sharp and focused even as you grow older? Having boundless energy and creativity to excel at work or in business? The ability to live it up every now and then and bounce back quickly? Or is it the fundamental state of being that allows you to get everything you want out of your life, including true happiness?

To me, good health means feeling at ease in my body, stable in my emotions, connected to the flow of life. It means having energy from the moment I wake up till the time I go to sleep. It means having clear skin, a well-functioning digestion, a toned body, a clear and calm mind. It means being able to do everything I want to do: travel, work, be there for my children, feel good, look good. Fifteen years ago, I was nowhere near this ideal picture. I couldn't get out of bed, felt depleted of energy most of the day, I was emotionally all over the place. I will do everything I need to never go back to that state. I am happy and don't think I could have ever felt this way with a body that was so out of order.

Health manifests in different ways and defining what is important to you is the first and most crucial step in creating wellness, as I discussed in chapter 1. And once you have this figured out and you set your eyes on this long-term goal, you will no longer think of living healthy as restrictive or boring. You will find it transformative. You will find great pleasure in looking good and feeling great and using that strength, resilience, mental stability, and energy to move forward on your path of self-actualisation.

What it ultimately comes down to is a decision: are you going to do the things that help you to become more of who you are meant to be and realising your fullest potential or are you going to do things that may hold you back – like consistently eating a crappy diet, over drinking, over eating, and ignoring your lack of sleep and stress levels.

Myth 2: It's all part of a plan

My grandfather smoked a packet of no-filter cigarettes and drank a glass of cognac every day. He ate bread for breakfast and lunch, and dinner was meat, potatoes, and vegetables. He lived till he was 85 and died of natural causes, no major illness.

I used to wonder what it was that allowed him to do all the things we now consider to be unhealthy, yet without an obvious ripple effect on his health. I am now sure it wasn't all about his diet. He was a man who lived a very active life, grew up in a time when food was simple, unprocessed, local, and seasonal. He spent his life in the exact same place that he was born and much of it outdoors. He also didn't know the word stress.

You could take his example as a sign that we have very little to say about our life. That it is all predestined, written in the cards and that it is all part of a plan. That we may as well enjoy ourselves and make the most out of our lives and throw caution to the wind, because hey, whatever happens is meant to happen. Except, you're not going to feel that way when you are diagnosed with a serious health condition.

Relying on destiny alone is a dangerous strategy. Even if you are doing fine today, you would want to avoid future health issues that have the potential to significantly impact the quality of your life or lead you on a long path of declining health that involves medication, hospitalisation, and treatments.

A better strategy is prevention. As I discussed in the previous chapter, the world has changed. We need to arm ourselves against the environmental influences that interfere with our ability to be our best. And this means doing the work to find out how to support yourself in the best way possible. It is not a 100% foolproof method because sometimes things still happen without obvious reason or explanation. But it makes sense to do what is within your power to set yourself up for success.

Myth 3: There are shortcuts

Who doesn't like a quick fix or a magic bullet? Advertising strategies are often created to tap into this desire: purchase our product and your happiness is guaranteed: you will look beautiful, your spouse will love you, you will feel energised. The world of health and wellness is no exception. Companies and individuals promote a certain diet, supplement, intervention, app, and make you think it is going to be the answer to all your problems. Examples of popular interventions in the world of health and longevity right now are IV vitamin infusions and anti-aging supplements.

What people fail to note is that the health benefits these expert biohackers are achieving are not just a result of supplementation. They have crafted their diet and lifestyle habits very carefully to build a strong foundation that allows additional interventions to enhance their effects. To use an analogy: they know they must tend the soil so that the high-quality seeds that they are planting are going to take root and grow into their full potential.

It is impossible to optimise your health and your life by focusing on just one thing and bypassing the creation of a strong foundation. Everything matters: what you eat, how you move, how you talk to yourself, your relationships, your stress levels, the quality of your sleep, your connection to something bigger than yourself, and your environment all influence how well you feel.

Everything is also connected: your thoughts impact your physical body; your physical body impacts your thoughts. You are a complex being and everything in this perfectly designed structure called your body-mind is interconnected. You can't hope to address a single area and ignore all the others. Full and complete health optimisation requires you address all the imbalances that exist. If you think you can short-cut your way out of this, think again. There isn't a supplement or IV vitamin infusion that can take the place of a healthy diet and lifestyle.

—◆—

CHAPTER 5

KNOW WHO YOU ARE

The 3 elements

To achieve anything, you need to have three things in place. You need to have the vision and goals as we talked about in chapter 1, and you need to have the skills to reach these goals. Skills can be learnt, and in the second half of the book I will impart my knowledge and the process that you can follow for your own journey.

For the specific goal that you are pursuing with the help of this book, which is health- and self-optimisation, you need a third thing: you need to become an expert on yourself. You need to understand your strengths and weaknesses, and what you need at any point in time to get the most out of you.

The most successful entrepreneurs in the world will tell you that their success doesn't happen by chance. It is a result of focus, commitment, learning, and putting in the work. Health-optimisation works in the same way. Before sharing the process and the steps for self-optimisation, let's look at what exactly it is that you are going to optimise. If you want to enhance your performance, your energy, your productivity, your focus, and your happiness you need to first understand: who are you?

I thought I knew myself pretty well. I knew what I liked and what I didn't, what made me feel good and what didn't. I just didn't always know why it was that way. I also didn't quite understand why I was so sensitive to certain foods, why my skin was always dry, why I didn't respond well to stress. I just accepted these things as being me. And then I started feeling suboptimal, could not find a medical explanation, and all of it became very confusing. Suddenly, it felt as if I was no longer in charge of my body. Whatever I tried, my body just didn't respond the way I thought it would. I was forced to look deeper to understand why I was struggling with my health and what was keeping me from feeling my best.

The subsequent health optimisation journey was, in a way, a journey of self-discovery. It was a gradual unpacking, peeling back the layers of an onion bit by bit until I figured out the reasons and the answers, and I learnt how to support myself in a way that allowed my body to function like a well-oiled machine.

This self-discovery process had many parts to it. It involved testing to identify underlying imbalances and inherent strengths and weaknesses. It involved trying things and tracking to see how I responded. I learnt how to connect parts of my life story to the onset of my symptoms, and this then provided clues as to what may be going on. Over time I learnt how to correct my imbalances and what I needed to put in place to feel my best. This involved optimising my diet, and using food to heal my gut and support my immune system. I needed to use supplements to correct some of the imbalances and I had to address lifestyle factors, such as stress management, movement, and exercise.

I also learnt that "I" was a complex being. I was a physical body-mind structure, one that was influenced by my genes and the interplay of these genes with the environment throughout my lifetime. What I am today is the result of the accumulation of experiences and influences. I learnt that this body-mind structure housed an entire ecosystem of microbes that are there to support my biology. That ecosystem had been heavily impacted over the entire course of my lifetime. And then there was the part of me that was intangible: the essence that powers up my being, breathing life into me and everything else in the universe. And I learnt how to harness this life force to be my best.

We are all a unique combination of these elements: our physical self, our microbial self, and the environment that we live in. The way these elements interact results in the unique package that is you. And all this needs to be looked at when working to achieve your highest potential.

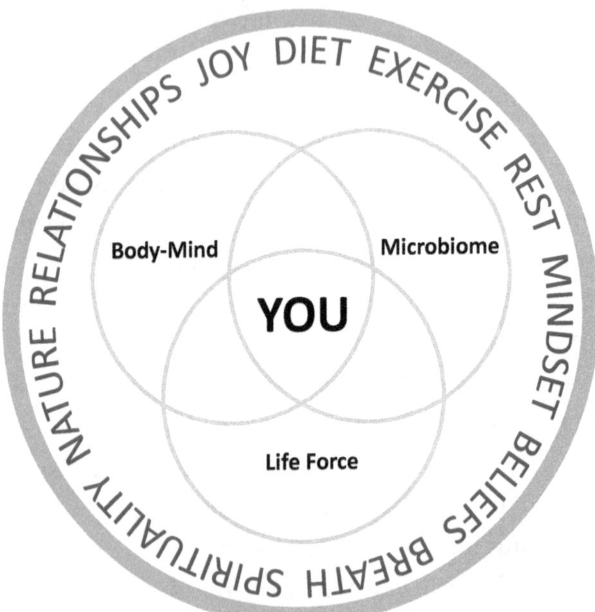

Your physical self

Who are you? This is a philosophical question that the greatest thinkers in history have been trying to answer. Rather than to get too philosophical about it, let's for a moment just consider this question from a purely physical perspective. Your "self", or the vehicle you inhabit is your body-mind, made up of cells, tissues, organs – a magnificent piece of creation that works seamlessly to keep your heart pumping, your lungs breathing, neurons firing, your cells signalling, your digestive system breaking down and absorbing food and so on. All of this without much conscious effort on your part. The complexity and efficiency of it all is truly amazing.

You inherited your unique genetic code from both of your parents at birth. And as your life progressed, the interaction of your genes and the environment helped to shape you into this unique body-mind that is you today.

To understand your physical self, in a personalised healthcare approach we spend a lot of time mapping out a person's life and health history. We draw up a detailed timeline that documents your family history: are there any illnesses or health conditions that could have been passed on genetically? We also look at your journey: what has happened during your life: the health of your parents at conception, your birth, childhood illnesses, life events, illnesses, stress, or trauma. What was your diet like as a child, as a teenager, as an adult? Are there any health issues that you experienced once or that are, perhaps, recurring?

When I examined my own life in this detailed manner, I was able to pinpoint several important factors that had impacted my journey: as a child I had recurring tonsillitis, skin eczema, allergies, and frequent ear infections, and numerous courses of antibiotics that undoubtedly altered my gut microbiome. I was prescribed a special birth control pill for teenage acne. When I moved to India I had a few very bad cases of gastroenteritis in quick succession, all of which were treated with antibiotics. Just by looking at these events it became clear that many of my health issues were connected to compromised gut health.

In a similar fashion, one of my clients, Alicia, a young and bubbly mompreneur, had been dealing with extreme acid reflux for a few years now. She walked up to me after a presentation that I did in my sons' school in Manila and told me she had come specially to hear my talk on gut health. "I have tried everything possible," she told me. "I have seen doctors who have done tests, prescribed medication for GERD (gastro-oesophageal reflux disease), I have tried natural supplements, eliminating foods from my diet and none of it has helped. I can't sleep at night because of the acidity, and I feel tired all the time. The one thing I need is energy with my small children and a business to run." It was clear that Alicia's digestive issues really affected her life and that she was at her wit's end.

She became a client, and I took her through the steps to help her find her solution. Alicia was already eating a clean and healthy diet, so I focused on gathering information to better understand her and determine the most appropriate short-term therapeutic diet and lifestyle approach. I drew up her health history and timeline with the help of a detailed questionnaire and then sat down to talk to her in more detail. I asked her to think back about the time she had started experiencing her symptoms: was there anything going on at that time? What did she remember?

When I asked her these questions Alicia thought for a moment and suddenly remembered that she had a severe bout of food poisoning while on holiday in Malaysia a few years prior. Not too long after that her digestive symptoms had started, getting progressively worse over time. This was an important clue: it is not uncommon for a bout of gastroenteritis to leave a lingering mark by creating microbial imbalances that don't automatically correct themselves. These microbial imbalances result in gut inflammation, a higher load of toxins, and changes in digestive function.

We focused on a short dietary reset to reduce her symptoms and allow the gut to heal and repair itself, brought in special supplements to restore gut barrier health and rebalance the microbiome. Alicia incorporated certain breathing practices to help with stress, sleep, and gut motility. After three months of doing the work, she no longer had any reflux symptoms and felt fantastic, and we then proceeded to move into a balanced and sustainable way of eating to keep her gut and body happy.

Insights from your genes

In 2007 scientists embarked on an ambitious project to map the human genome. The result of this project brought us a lot of insights and new knowledge. We discovered that what makes us unique is the individual gene variants and more importantly, that these genetic variants are "malleable". One of the greatest insights of the human genome studies has been that your genes are not your destiny but that our environment can influence gene expression. This concept is also known as epigenetics. Genes can be switched on and switched off and the factors that contribute to this process are environmental factors that are very often within our control.

The mechanisms that influence gene expression respond to a wide variety of triggers, ranging from the food we eat, stress, exercise, exposure to environmental toxins, our emotions, and cues from our "microbial self" (more on that later). This is an important concept because it gives us a certain level of control over the way our life progresses.

Within the context of knowing your "self" so that you can better support yourself in the best way possible, it can be helpful to look at your unique genetic strengths and weaknesses. Examining your family history is one way of capturing relevant genetic information. Using nutrigenetic testing is another way to identify the presence of genetic variants that can have a potential impact on the way your body functions, like your metabolism, blood sugar regulation, and detoxification. There are many variants that have good research evidence for the potential of diet and lifestyle factors to positively modify their expression. These tests should always be looked at within the context of your current health and your symptoms. I will discuss testing in more detail in chapter 11.

Your microbial self

A few years after the start of the human genome project in 2007, the United States National Institute of Health launched the Human Microbiome Project to better understand the role of microbiota in human health and disease. Scientists understood that we had a staggering number of microbes that lived in and on our human bodies, but they did not know a lot about the impact of these microbes on our biological functions.

Mind-boggling discoveries ensued and revealed that we are not just human – we are a living and breathing ecosystem or, as some scientists have pointed out, a walking column of microbes. Over 100 trillion microbial cells inhabit our bodies and directly affect our health and disease. These micro-organisms influence our energy levels, our hormones, they talk to our brain, regulate our appetite, synthesise nutrients and, when out of balance, contribute to everything from obesity to chronic fatigue and brain fog.

Since the birth of modern medicine, the attention has been on the impact of our human genes on health and disease. The relatively recent discovery of the microbiome, which is the collective genetic material of our own resident micro-organisms, has revealed that our own genes are just a small part of what influences our health. While we possess about 22,000 genes, the microbiome is thought to have 200 times the number of genes. Collectively, your microbiome influences a large part of your biology.

While there is still a lot we don't know about the microbiome, it is clear that we need to support this inner ecosystem in the best way we can. The delicate balance between the different microbes is easily influenced by environmental factors such as toxins, the wrong foods, stress, and medication. Imbalances are linked to many health issues ranging from obesity to chronic fatigue, autoimmune conditions, anxiety, depression, and brain fog. There are now ways to analyse parts of the microbiome, for example, the gut or the oral microbiome, with specialised tests that look at the composition of your gut microbes as well as the gastrointestinal environment. It was such a test that helped me to identify the main root cause of my health issues. My test results showed that my gut microbiome was out of balance. I had unwanted microbes, a lack of beneficial bacteria, and the gastro-intestinal environment that these micro-organisms resided in had metaphorical holes in the roof and toxins floating around. My microbial-self, which was supposed to support my health, had, instead, been sabotaging my success.

In the many years that followed these findings it became clear that many (if not all) of my symptoms resulted from this compromised gut and microbiome: from my fatigue, mood swings, hormonal imbalances to skin issues. With targeted nutrition, supplement, and lifestyle changes I was able to restore my gut, get rid of the bad players, strengthen my digestion, and resolve all my issues. The results were truly amazing. My skin cleared up, my digestion settled down, I was able to eat everything again without having food reactions, and I had plenty of energy and felt calm and balanced.

It also became clear that most of my clients' symptoms were in some way connected to imbalances in their microbiome and the environment that these microbes lived in. Even symptoms that were seemingly unrelated to their digestion. By addressing these imbalances, the same clients managed to get rid of anxiety attacks, heart palpitations, aches and pains, and skin issues. Their sleep became deep and restful, their energy levels increased, and they had a more positive outlook on life.

To optimise your health and your life, you must optimise all of you: your physical self and your microbial self: the collective community of microbes that play an essential role in your wellbeing. How you do that I will cover in the next part of the book. First, let's look at one more element that requires attention if we want to fully optimise our lives.

Your life force

You have a physical body, a mind, and microbes that help support the functioning of this body-mind. And then there is a more intangible force that breathes life into you the moment you are born and that leaves your body when you die. Some call it your soul, others consciousness or spirit. Life force is the term I love the most – it is the essence of life, yours and everyone and everything else that exists. Incomprehensible and intangible, yet there are moments when you experience its true beauty: in moments where you feel what are called sublime emotions, like deep love, happiness, bliss, or awe. You feel the connection to this life force when you are purely present in the moment, free from any thoughts and you are fully immersed in the here and now.

Unlike the physical body-mind or our microbial non-self, we can't manipulate or alter or correct this life force. But, to live our life to our fullest potential we can learn to connect with it. Allow it to guide us. Practices like meditation, breathing or yoga bring us in connection with that part of ourselves. Learning to live mindfully has the same result. In the next section of the book, I will share some powerful tools that help you to be more present, grounded, and connected to your life force.

Environmental inputs

You exist within an environment that provides you continuous inputs throughout your lifetime. Some of these inputs are within your control, like your diet and lifestyle choices. Some are not. You may be or have been exposed to environmental toxins, physical or psychological trauma, radiation, micro-organisms like viruses, bacteria, or parasites. All these exposures impact your physical and mental self, your thoughts, beliefs, gene expression, and physiological processes. It impacts your non-self by changing the microbial balance. And it impacts your connection with your life force.

In a personalised health optimisation approach, you, therefore, start with the environment first. While you can't change what has already happened in your lifetime, you can change your current environment and become aware of how your past environment has impacted your health and wellbeing and use that information to correct the current inputs.

With this understanding, allow me to take you through the process of optimising you.

PART 2

THE PERSONALISED PATH

In the next few chapters, I am going to take you through the steps that I follow when taking a client through a personalised health optimisation journey. These steps are:

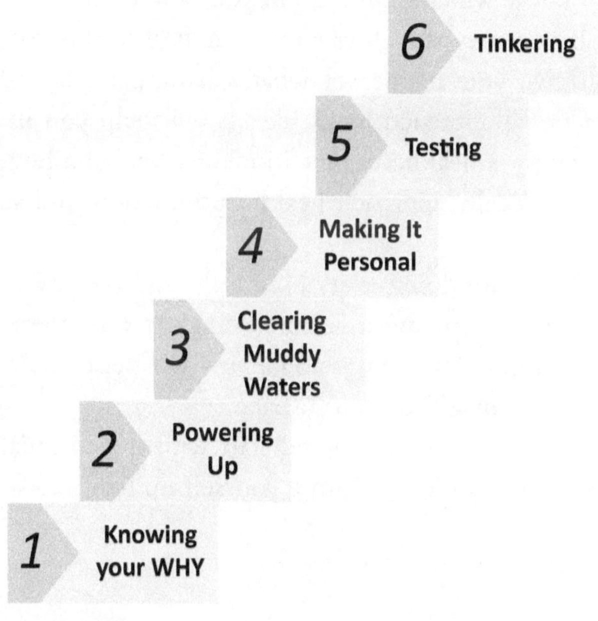

There are a few things I should mention before you dive in. The very fact that health is personal means that this book won't be able to give you all your answers. The second important point is that the world of health and wellness is rapidly evolving. There are new apps and technologies continuously appearing on the scene. It is impossible to include everything in this book. What the next few chapters will give you is a roadmap that you can follow. You can use this roadmap to assess where you are, and where your focus should be. Wherever you are on your journey, there are always steps you can take to support your health. While reading through the steps, you will know which ones require your attention.

If you are struggling with your health, this roadmap will give you an idea of what a truly personalised and functional approach looks like. It will help you in your search for a healthcare practitioner by knowing how they should ideally approach health optimisation in a similar fashion.

If you are doing everything right and you are feeling great, keep doing what you are doing! And use these steps as a reminder or as a way to identify what else you can do to keep yourself in tip top shape.

And now, let's dig in and start with the essential first step on this journey: setting yourself up for success.

CHAPTER 6

KNOWING YOUR WHY

In the first part of the book, I talked about the importance of having a vision for yourself. If you don't know where you are going, you are never going to get there. So, what you are going to have to do first is evaluate what you are trying to change, what will be the outcome of that change process, and what the success factors are that you need to put in place before you begin.

Key questions

It took quite a long time before I reached a point in my own life where I had no choice in my mind but to do what needed to be done to feel better. I was, as I like to say, at that point where I knew "this couldn't go on."

I regularly have conversations with people who are struggling with health issues, and I take them through a set of questions that make them really stop and think about how that health issue is affecting their life and potentially their future. This is a powerful way to shift from "I know I have this issue but otherwise I am fine" to "this can't go on because if it does, it will impact my life and my future."

When I first spoke to Helena, she told me she had suffered from Irritable Bowel Syndrome (IBS) for many years. IBS affects between 7 to 21 % of the population and is characterised by gastrointestinal symptoms such as abdominal pain and discomfort, diarrhoea, constipation, or both. When she was originally diagnosed, after a tedious process of testing for other gastrointestinal diseases, doctors had told her that there wasn't anything she could do about it and so she had learnt to live with the pain and the discomfort. She had recently read somewhere that IBS could be cured naturally, with dietary changes, and this was one of the reasons Helena had reached out to me. She wanted to see if I could help. To get a better understanding of what was going on I asked her this question: besides the digestive issues, if she had a magic wand, what would she use it for to change in her life?

Helena thought for a moment and then starting talking. She and her partner were ready for a baby and lately she had been experiencing terrible mood swings and her partner had been on the receiving end of these. She realised it wasn't fair on him but more importantly, she wondered how she was going to be able to be a good mom if she snapped at the drop of a hat, going from happy to angry to sad without being able to control it? She said: "I want to be the healthiest I can be for myself, my partner, who I love and who is so supportive, and I want to be the best mom I can be and for that I need to feel calm and balanced and in control." Helena had IBS and had accepted stomach pains, diarrhoea, and bloating for many years but it was her mood swings that were impacting her life the most.

I asked her what she thought would happen if she wasn't able to get this sorted and she shuddered as she imagined being on that emotional rollercoaster forever and the impact it would have on the people she loved the most. When I asked her what she could see happen if she did get this sorted, she smiled as she imagined feeling balanced and strong and having a most beautiful life with her partner and children. Helena had uncovered the real reason for embarking on a health optimisation journey.

We don't often stop to think about consequences. Most of us are optimists when it comes to our health: we believe that our bodies are resilient and capable, that we are invincible. We live with our heads in the cloud, thinking everything will be fine. Even if around us people are diagnosed with cancer, dying from heart attacks, or are hobbling along with multiple symptoms. A reality check can be a powerful way to create some perspective and to get inspired to make changes.

At the end of this book you will find a symptom questionnaire. Use it to honestly highlight the things that are currently out of balance in your body. Then come back to answer the following questions:

1. If you had a magic wand and you could change anything you wanted about your current health, what would you change?
2. If you didn't do anything about these symptoms, what do you think would happen?
3. What, on the other hand, would happen if you got this under control?

Your deepest why

You are reading this book because you decided, at some point, to take your health and your life seriously. You have chosen to participate actively in the creation of optimal health and wellbeing. As I explained in chapter 2, the choice you have made is not an easy one; it takes commitment, focus, and a willingness to engage in battle against the current norm. Society in general will not offer you support. In fact, it may even try to sabotage your efforts. You will find the very foods that you are trying to eliminate lurking in every possible corner: in the grocery store, in commercials, at parties, lunches, cafés, restaurants, and at your friend's house. People may raise their eyebrows and question your sanity. They will feel threatened and judged when you decline to eat what they eat.

You are going to defy what is normal, battle against the status quo, and this requires dedication, effort, and commitment. And therefore, in addition to answering the key questions, you have to spend some time getting really clear on your motivating factors, your outcome and your vision for yourself. So that you are firmly rooted in the reasons for taking on this journey.

Diane came to work with me because she was dealing with digestive issues, in particular, severe bloating, uncontrollable sugar cravings, and brain fog. Although her immediate motivation was to resolve these symptoms, we spent some time analysing her bigger "why" and it didn't take her very long to formulate this: her mother was suffering from Alzheimer's and watching her cognitive decline gave Diane a very clear and specific motivation to do whatever was required to avoid a similar path. She was determined to spare her own children from having to deal with this. In Diane's words: "I want to be 80 years old and have the ability to go for a hike with my children, not have them come to a nursing home to visit whatever is 'left of me'. I want to be able to live my life to the fullest with a quick and steep decline at the very end, rather than years of gradual suffering."

Whether Diane's story resonates with you or whether your ultimate motivating factor is to have energy and focus to fulfil your unique dreams and purpose, it is important to get clear on this. So, complete the goal exercise below and define your ultimate vision and outcome. Define what is worthwhile enough for you to be making consistent effort. Be as specific as you can be and think about what keeps tugging at your heart. Uncover your deepest dreams and desires and think about how being in optimal health will help you manifest the vision you have for yourself. Write this all out and keep it somewhere close, where you can see it.

Question 1: What are your immediate health goals and intentions for embarking on this journey? What do you want to be different after one month, three months, one year from today?

Question 2: What is the real reason behind the changes you seek in your life? What is your biggest WHY? – think about what is going to change in your life when you reach these goals. Why is this important to you? What will your life look and feel like?

Think of the things you love about your life, and the things you don't. Think about what keeps tugging at your heart. For example: feeling more confident and comfortable in your skin, taking your career to the next level, finding the drive and confidence to set up your own business, re-kindling your marriage, being a better parent, bringing back the joy in your life, finding your passion so that you can give your life direction and meaning, etc. Imagine what it would feel or look like when your dreams have come true – who would you be, where would you live, what would you have created?

Success factors

My most successful clients have set up a support system that ensures they are geared up for success. They have created a network of professionals around them to turn to for help when needed: a trusted doctor, personal trainer, yoga teacher, chiropractor, massage therapist, coach, and any other wellness professional that can help keep them on track. And they have the support of family members or friends.

Aaron, a corporate executive client who had a very demanding job and symptoms that were interfering with his ability to do his job properly, asked me for the fastest possible solution. The strategy I created for him included a short period of a therapeutic healing diet that eliminated several foods. He followed it diligently and managed to turn his health around quite quickly. Much of his success had to do with the support of his wife, who used my nutrition guidelines to create healthy and delicious meals for him to have at home and take to office.

This kind of support on the home front is often what makes or breaks a health optimisation process. And even if you don't have someone to cook for you, you can consider roping in a friend to help you with accountability. Some of my clients use a high-quality food delivery service for a short while to support their dietary requirements. If you surround yourself with individuals who are on a similar path as you, who value their health and make choices that support their health goals, you are more likely to succeed. Additionally, ask yourself what else will keep you inspired. Here are some key questions that you can use to identify which success factors you need to put in place to lay a strong and unbreakable foundation.

- What kind of support do you need to make this journey a success? (e.g. accountability, shopping, meal preparation, inspiration)
- Who in your life can offer this kind of support? (e.g. your spouse, mother, child, friend or colleague)
- What changes are required in your daily routine?

CHAPTER 7

POWERING UP

2 Powering Up

Many years of doing this work with clients have made me realise that there is a common practice that results in a higher chance of success in achieving goals. And it is not only my clients; most highly productive people use a similar approach to drive their success.

I call it the Mindful Morning Routine. Based on three important pillars, this Mindful Morning Routine is akin to powering up your engine, supercharging your body and your mind at the start of your day, and getting into the right frame of mind for optimal performance.

A morning routine

We are continuously pulled into every direction by the responsibilities we have towards our family, friends, homes, careers, and other things. Only to lose track of ourselves in the process. And slowly, over time, we give in on our energy levels, our health, our looks, our inner balance, and our peace of mind, and taking care of all our responsibilities becomes more and more difficult.

Remember the safety instructions they give you on board of an airplane? In case of an emergency, place the oxygen mask over your own mouth and nose before helping the person sitting next to you. Why? Because you need to be taken care of, calm, and breathing before you can help someone else.

This rule applies to life in general. You are in a much better position to help others and look after your responsibilities if you are fit, energetic, calm, and balanced. And to get to that point you must invest some time in yourself. For yourself but also for the world that depends on you. It is not selfish. It is self-nurturing. You must put yourself first.

At some point in my life, I would hit the ground running. The alarm would go off and after dragging myself out of bed, it was go-go from the get-go. Children, school, work, husband, social engagements, housework, finances, homework, extracurricular activities, pets – I would keep on running until it was time to go to sleep. This is how days would just fly by. Many of my clients are in the same boat. And when we discuss incorporating some self-care practices, they tell me they just don't have the time. Here's the thing though: by carving out time, even if it feels impossible to do, you eventually reap the benefits.

When I started prioritising and taking some time in the morning to do the things that help me feel more peaceful, balanced, and connected, I started feeling more in charge of my life. I made better choices. I became more productive and focused. It felt as if I had more time instead of less.

I see the same benefits with my clients. The most successful ones make this a non-negotiable part of their day. Once it is an inherent part of your routine you notice the difference when you skip this more than a few days in a row.

Key elements

There are three elements that comprise a powerful Mindful Morning Routine: morning sunlight, a mindfulness practice, and a form of movement. I will list the benefits of each and how it contributes to health optimisation, as well as the many different options that are available to you. Remember that this is your personal path to wellness so you can completely make it your own.

Morning sunlight

Many of our body's biological processes are regulated by an internal body clock, also known as the circadian rhythm. This inner clock is located in your brain, in an area called the suprachiasmatic nucleus. This area guides a network of "sub" clocks that are housed throughout the body in various tissues and organs. Through this network our body goes through physical and mental changes according to a 24-hour cycle.

There are many external cues, also known as Zeitgebers (a German word for "time givers" or "synchronisers") that our internal body clocks respond to. Some examples are temperature, meal timings, exercise, social interaction, nutrition, and medicine, and one of the most important cues is the light/dark or day/night cycle of the earth.

As described in the first part of this book, we evolved over millions of years while being completely in tune with the cycles of nature. We would rise with the sun and sleep when the sun would set. By sensing morning daylight, our bodies naturally slow down the production of melatonin, which is a hormone that induces sleep, and it naturally increases the production of cortisol, the hormone that gets us up and going.

Nowadays we spend time indoors, much of it in artificial light, but exposing yourself to morning sunlight can help to regulate your body clock and set you up for an energised day and later on, a good night's sleep.

I like to spend my first 10 minutes of the day outside in my garden with a glass of warm water, watching the world around me wake up. If you live in an apartment, head out to the balcony, or open a window and get that early morning sunlight on your face. Or take the dog or yourself out for an early morning walk, which gives you the extra benefit of combining your morning sunlight with movement.

Movement

Movement and exercise have a tremendous amount of benefits. One of those is the boost in lymphatic circulation and the other one is the release of dopamine. Dopamine is the happy hormone. It makes you feel good. And it doesn't take much to trigger this process. Including a form of movement of choice in the morning will help to loosen up your muscles, boost circulation, activate your life force and get you in a happier state of mind, ready to tackle the day ahead.

There are many ways to approach this. You may choose to do a few functional movements like lunges, squats, push-ups, a few jumping jacks, stretching or your full workout routine. A morning walk or a run, some sun salutations – the choice is yours. Even if you are in the habit of exercising at a later part of the day, taking 10-15 minutes in the morning to add a bit of movement will make a noticeable difference.

I like to spend 15 minutes on most mornings to practice some Kundalini yoga. It combines physical movement with breathing and meditation and after those 15 minutes I am feeling awake, energised, limber, and grounded. A few days a week I do a full workout with HIIT and weight training, and on occasion when I have some more time, I may do a full Kundalini yoga practice.

You will have to find what works best for you –

remember it is personal – but do make this a habit and watch the impact it makes on your day.

Mindfulness practice

Before proceeding, I would like to ask you to take a moment and sit up with a straight spine, feet firmly planted on the ground and hands resting in your lap. Close your eyes and take a few deep breaths in through your nose, and out of your mouth. Then return to breathing normally and bring your awareness into your body. Consciously drop your shoulders and relax your muscles and notice how your feet are touching the floor, the weight of your hands on your legs. Shift your awareness to your breath, noticing the rising and falling of your belly, the cool air entering your nostrils and the touch of warm air on your upper lip as you exhale. Stay with this awareness for a few minutes before opening your eyes again.

What do you notice? This short little practice has probably made you feel more calm, relaxed, and present. On a biochemical level, you have shifted your nervous system into a parasympathetic state and on a mental level you are more attuned to your body and your environment. You are more mindful and aware and intuitive and connected to your life force and that is a wonderful, powerful state to be in.

I have spoken about our life force in previous chapters: that which infuses life into you, me, and the entire universe. We catch glimpses of this universal intelligence when we are present in the here and now. And that is what a mindfulness practice is helping you achieve: a deeper sense of connection and presence. All of that in a matter of a few minutes.

Imagine being this grounded and connected throughout your day. Imagine how calmly and clearly you will be making decisions, how present you will be when engaging with people, able to pick up on their state of mind. It is possible. It is a habit you can create and the process of creating this habit starts with a simple commitment to spend a few minutes every morning to cultivate this state of being.

You are not going to be able to sustain this state permanently, at least not at first. Everything around you is set up to distract you. Most of all, your phone and social media, and besides that life in general will demand your attention, often for multiple things at the same time. But a simple morning routine will remind you of what it feels like to be purely present and soon you will learn to shift back into this state periodically throughout your day. You will learn to be in charge of your life, rather than life being in charge of you.

40 days to creating new habits

Building new habits isn't an overnight thing. Who hasn't made a resolution to incorporate a new habit only to watch the commitment fizzle out after a few weeks or even days. Part of the reason for this is that we set the bar too high at the beginning. We enthusiastically embark on a challenging new practice that is just not feasible on an everyday basis. Which is why you want to decide on something simple – a minimum amount of time that you can afford to allocate to your new habit on even the busiest of days.

And that is why you want to aim for 15 minutes. Who doesn't have 15 minutes in the morning to practice this powerful routine? Start with just that. You can combine morning sunlight, mindfulness, and movement into one by going for a mindful walk or, as I do, spend 15 minutes on a short yoga routine outdoors that incorporates movement, breathing, and meditation.

According to the ancient science of yoga it takes 40 days to create a permanent habit. After doing something for 40 days, it becomes ingrained in your routine, much like taking a shower in the morning or brushing your teeth. You don't have to think about such habits, you just do them. What you want is to get to a stage where your Mindful Morning Routine habits are second nature. Even if you skip a day for whatever reason, you will fall back into the routine on the next day. To get to that stage, all you need to do is commit to 15 minutes for 40 days. Print out a calendar and start ticking off and watch how this simple strategy has the power to change your life.

CHAPTER 8

CLEARING THE MUDDY WATERS - FOOD FIRST

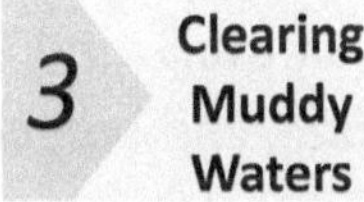

It is impossible to see the bottom of a pond or pool when there is mud floating around in the water. Only when the dirt settles are you able to get a clear view. The same principle applies to your health. To see what is going on and what is driving your symptoms, you need to first clear the muddy waters.

David reached out to me because he was worried about his health. David was an expat and a successful banker. In the past couple of months, he had experienced two episodes where his heart had started racing out of control and he felt out of breath. The experience had been very frightening and felt like he was having a heart attack. Both times he rushed to the emergency room and after being thoroughly checked and kept under supervision for the night, he was sent home with a clean bill of health. He continued to experience a sense of anxiety, and all of this was affecting his life and ability to perform at his job. He desperately wanted to know what was causing this and how he could support himself better to feel calm and in control.

A detailed look at David's health history, lifestyle, and diet habits showed that there were a lot of things in the mix: his diet was suboptimal as he had little time to prepare proper meals and ordered in most of his food. His food choices included a lot of quick and easy feel-good foods such as sandwiches, pizza, and burgers, and he had taken to drinking a few glasses of alcohol at the end of every day to take the edge off. He exercised a few times a week but was sedentary otherwise. He had struggled with gut issues almost his entire life and was regularly taking antacids to help control acid reflux. His job was very stressful, and he was working long hours, often ruminating about issues while trying to sleep at night.

After giving me this background, he asked, "Why do you think I have suddenly started feeling these regular bouts of anxiety? And what can I do to fix it?" I explained to him that anxiety can have several root causes. There can be a life event or situation that brings on anxiety but when you experience anxiety out of the blue, without any apparent reason, it is often brought on by imbalances in the body. Neurotransmitter imbalances, hormones, inflammation, impaired gut health, nutrient deficiencies, microbial imbalances can all be playing a role. To see what is really going on it is important to first clear the muddy waters. To take out all the potential culprits, which are the factors that are muddling things up. Then you can begin to see more clearly what the underlying root causes are and begin to address them.

What are these factors? They are the collective inputs from your environment. Examples are foods that are causing inflammation, empty calories that are filing you up but lacking important nutrients, foods that are irritating your digestive tract or that are triggering an immune response. It also includes toxins from your environment, stress, a lack of sleep or too much or too little exercise.

Clearing up your environment, streamlining your diet and lifestyle is a foundational and fundamental first step in the process of health optimisation. And it is often not given enough attention. Clearly not in a conventional medicine setting but also in functional or integrative healthcare approach there is often a tendency to move straight into costly root cause investigations before the foundation is put into place. Many of the clients I work with and help support in streamlining their diet and lifestyle see a remarkably quick resolution of their symptoms and often don't even need to take it to a next level of testing. You can't underestimate how important these factors are.

So, let's have a look at what it means to be clearing

the muddy waters, starting with the general baseline principles that form the foundation for a healthy diet. The next chapter will cover clearing up the muddy waters from a lifestyle perspective.

Food first – Know the basics

Some of the culprits that are contributing to your muddy waters are unique to you. I will talk about these personal factors in chapter 10 but first, I will take you through the **basic** principles of a healthy diet. Principles that apply to everyone and that should form the baseline approach. You may already be following these principles, in which case, feel free to skim through this and treat it as a reminder. If you are not already following these principles, doing so will help you to start feeling better and clear some of the symptoms you are dealing with.

My core principles of a healthy diet are inspired by Michael Pollan. Michael Pollan is an American author and journalist who has written extensively about a variety of subjects including nutrition. His book "Food Rules" outlines and explains the simple but powerful fundamental principles of a healthy diet: **Eat food. Mostly plants. Not too much.**

Let's unpack that.

Principle 1: Eat (real) food

Real, whole foods are natural, fresh foods that are unrefined and unprocessed. They are full and complete packages of nutrients in perfect balance, the way nature intended them to be. Any food that has had a part of it removed lacks a natural balance of nutrients and often the body starts craving that missing part. For example, refined white flour lacks important nutrients and the fibre we badly need. Processed foods are typically made in factories, come in boxes or bags, and have long lists of ingredients, some of which are manmade and hard to recognise.

When choosing what to eat, you want to choose food that is **real**, **traditional**, and **wholesome**. You should be able to look at the food on your plate, recognise the ingredients, and imagine in your mind's eye where they came from and how they got here.

Principle 2: Mostly plants

Whether your body loves animal protein or whether you are a vegetarian, plant foods are a critical component of your diet. Plant foods include vegetables, fruits, nuts and seeds, whole grains, and legumes. In general (and I will talk in more detail about personalisation in chapter 10), you want to include a range of rainbow-coloured vegetables in every meal and eat a few portions of fruit daily. This is what supplies your body with most of its nutrients in the form of vitamins and minerals, fibre, antioxidants, as well as plant-based nutrients.

All these nutrients are essential for our bodies to build and maintain a strong immune system and provide the co-factors for detoxification and cellular repair mechanisms, all of which help to protect us from chronic disease. Additionally, the fibre in whole plant foods keeps our digestive system healthy, along with other plant compounds such as polyphenols that feed the beneficial bacteria in our gut, thereby helping to build a balanced and diverse microbiome. As I explained in chapter 6, your gut microbiome, aka your microbial self, plays a critical role in your health and a diverse population of gut microbes is an important marker of good health.

If plants don't currently have a prominent place in your diet, begin by including more (5 to 7 portions a day) of rainbow-coloured vegetables in your diet. This is a perfect way to start crowding out unhealthy foods and to begin noticing an instant increase in energy.

Principle 3: Not too much

Overeating, as well as unlimited snacking between meals, contributes to health problems and interferes with proper digestion and blood sugar regulation. There is a growing body of evidence for the health benefits that result from incorporating periods of fasting and periods of caloric restriction. Without going into too much detail on the science of fasting, the consensus is that creating space between meals is part of the "not too much" diet principle.

This is also where it becomes important to slow down and eat your meals slowly, with awareness and in a relaxed setting. To chew your food properly, savour the taste, and recognise when you have had enough. To wait a few hours before you eat again so that your digestive system can complete its job, uninterrupted. To leave at least 12 hours between your dinner and breakfast to reap the benefits of an overnight fasting period.

When making food choices, ask yourself:

"Is this real, whole food?

Do I recognise the ingredients?

Has it been minimally processed?"

"Am I adding to my ideal daily portions of fresh vegetables and fruits?"

"Am I taking the time to enjoy and really taste my food?"

"Have I had enough or am I eating for the sake of eating?"

These are straightforward principles but if adhered to consistently, they are very powerful. If you follow these principles every time you choose to eat something you are well on your way to becoming a much healthier version of yourself.

Putting the principles into practice

This next section may be common sense, but I do want to highlight the main categories of foods that don't belong in a healthy diet. These are foods that contribute to inflammation and all other health conditions that are connected to this and that form the empty calories that are keeping your body deprived of essential nutrients.

- **Refined / processed and artificial foods** (such as soda, biscuits, cookies, chips, candy, juices, white flour, refined grains, etc.)

  This category includes foods that come in packages, plastic, boxes and containers and that have an endless list of ingredients, most of which you can't even recognise. These are also foods that have been stripped of their natural goodness, such as refined flours and everything that is made with it.

- **Refined vegetable seed oils**

  This category includes all the inflammatory oils that have been extracted from seeds like corn, sunflower, canola, soy, grape seeds, and cottonseeds.

- **(Refined) Sugar**

  To summarise, an overload of sugar or refined carbohydrates can result in a wide variety of imbalances, including blood sugar imbalances (leading to energy fluctuations and mood swings), insulin resistance, weight gain, cardiovascular disease, systemic inflammation, thyroid issues, mineral depletion, reduced immune function, compromised brain function, yeast overgrowth and other microbial imbalances, and reduced oral health.

The above listed foods are not good for anyone. Without exception, everyone will reap the benefits of eliminating these from their diet. There is a second category of foods: foods that are tolerated by some but, in my experience as well as based on research, very often contribute to health issues. These foods are gluten and dairy. In my practice I find that eliminating this second category of foods always speeds up the healing process by giving the digestive system and the immune system a break. You may think these foods are fine for you, and maybe that is indeed the case. But you may also be surprised to see how you feel without them.

The way to find out whether they are a problem for you is to strictly remove them from your diet for a particular period and take note of how you feel. I usually recommend 30 days, after which you can reintroduce them one by one to see how your body responds.

Let's have a quick look at what these foods are and the reasons they may be detrimental to your health.

- **Gluten**
  Global awareness of the potential issues related to gluten has increased, especially with respect to Celiac Disease, which is the most severe level of gluten intolerance. What many people (including doctors) still don't fully understand is that Celiac Disease is only the tip of the iceberg. For every Celiac patient there are many more people that suffer from lower levels of gluten sensitivity which stay undiagnosed. Adding to the problem is the fact that gluten related

symptoms are not limited to digestive issues and can show up in countless other different ways.

You may wonder why gluten related issues are increasing in prevalence. There are a few reasons for that. From a human evolution perspective, grains are a relatively "recent" addition to our diets. They were added approximately 10,000 years ago when the shift happened from a hunter-gatherer lifestyle to an agricultural lifestyle. Grains, including wheat, provide us with all the major nutrient groups that our bodies need: carbohydrates, protein, fats, vitamins, minerals, and fibre, and it is, therefore, not difficult to understand that grains have been an important and popular dietary component. There are, however, a few potential problems associated with grain consumption.

Grains contain certain compounds that can interfere with digestion. The most well-known example of this is gluten, which is found in wheat as well as some other grains, such as rye, barley, spelt, and triticale. Once gluten enters our bodies, it is broken down by digestive enzymes into peptides. Some of these gluten peptides can trigger an immune response. When there is a non-stop supply of gluten coming into our digestive track it can result in continuous inflammation in the gut, an out-of-control immune system, and eventually different kinds of health problems. And it doesn't help that most of us already have an impaired immune system as well as a compromised digestive system due to factors such as stress, poor diet, and over-use of antibiotics.

To top it all, the wheat we eat today is very different from the wheat that was grown many years ago. Through genetic modification scientists have been able to cultivate higher-yielding crops that have lower mineral content, higher gluten content, and a different kind of gluten protein which a majority of people with Celiac Disease react negatively to. All of the above factors are major contributors to the rise in gluten and wheat allergies and sensitivities world over.

- **Dairy**
  There are several problems linked with the consumption of milk and other dairy products. In short:
  - Off-the-shelf milk is factory farmed and contains growth hormones and antibiotics.
  - The process of pasteurisation and homogenisation alters the chemical structure of milk, which makes it difficult to digest.
  - Many adults don't make the enzyme lactase, which is required to digest the lactose in milk.
  - The combination of lactose and whey causes insulin spikes.

Because of these problems, the consumption of dairy products can contribute to digestive issues, hormonal imbalances, and insulin resistance, all of which in turn contribute to the inflammatory process in your body.

There are, of course, forms of dairy that are easier to digest (such as fermented dairy or raw dairy), and dairy which is obtained from grass-fed cows, free of hormones and antibiotics. For people who can tolerate and digest dairy, this can be a very nutrient dense and healthy part of a diet. However, as with gluten, to identify if dairy is good for you, I recommend eliminating it for a period followed by a reintroduction challenge with clean dairy forms to see how you respond.

What you should eat

To summarise, to clean up your diet you want to move to a wholefoods-based diet that is free from the foods outlined above and that contains

- plenty (aim for 7 portions a day) of colourful non-starchy vegetables
- healthy fats (like extra virgin olive oil, coconut oil, ghee)
- protein (like eggs, chicken, fish, seafood, meat, some dairy if tolerated)
- some starchy vegetables (like potatoes, sweet potatoes, and other root vegetables like carrot, beetroot, squash)
- fruits
- nuts and seeds
- beans and legumes
- spices and herbs
- whole grains.

There are a few additional factors that are important to consider in this first phase.

- **Go local**
  The freshest produce is grown near your home. It has taken only a short amount of time to get to where you shop and is, therefore, fresher, has more nutrients, and tastes better. And let's not forget the positive impact of eating locally grown produce on your local economy and on your carbon footprint.

- **Eat seasonal**
  Different fruits and vegetables grow in different seasons, and they are perfectly designed to support our health accordingly. Root vegetables give us warmth and grounding in the colder winter months, melons and squashes are cooling in the summer, and young green salad leaves help support the transition between these two seasons in the springtime by helping to support the detoxification processes in our body. Try, as much as possible, to live in harmony with the cycles and rhythm of nature.

- **Choose organic where possible**
  It is important to do what we can to reduce our exposure to toxins. One place to start is by choosing organic produce when you can. It reduces your intake of pesticides, toxins, and other harmful chemicals. If you are not in a position to buy everything organic, start by having a look at the "dirty dozen" – a list of

vegetables and fruits that tend to have the highest amount of pesticides and begin there.

- **Quality matters**

When choosing your animal protein, it is important to keep into consideration where it came from, if the animal was raised under humane and natural conditions, and if it was fed a diet that it was genetically meant to be eating. For example, a cow needs to be allowed to roam around the fields and graze on grass. A chicken is supposed to run around freely and eat a natural diet of worms, insects and be allowed to lay its eggs freely. Fish should be sustainably farmed or caught without the use of common questionable industry practices. Choose smaller fish over larger ones to reduce mercury exposure.

- **Hydration**

Water is what keeps our cells, tissues, organs, joints, etc. functioning properly. It is essential for maintaining a stable body temperature, for waste removal, joint lubrication, digestion of food and more. Dehydration leads to feeling thirsty (which is often mistaken for hunger), it causes fatigue, nausea, headaches, and when dehydration is chronic there are many more serious potential side effects. A general guideline is eight glasses of water a day but how much water you need exactly depends on many factors such as your physical activity level, the climate you live in, your diet, and stress levels.

I want to reiterate that the above outlined diet principles are general principles. If you have been eating a diet that contains a lot of inflammatory, processed, and refined foods, if your diet has been lacking in essential fibre or colourful plant foods, you will experience a tremendous beneficial shift by incorporating these general principles alone. If your diet has been healthy, but it has a lot of dairy and gluten and you feel suboptimal in any way, you can experiment by eliminating these two categories of food.

For some people these general and foundational nutrition principles are enough to bring about better health and balance. If despite eating according to these principles you still feel suboptimal or have health symptoms of any kind, it is time to take it to the next phase of your personalised health optimisation process.

As I alluded to in previous chapters, we are all unique and it's all personal. We have our unique stories, circumstances, health challenges, genetics, gut microbiomes, and experiences that will inform a more targeted and personalised approach to our diet and lifestyle. In chapter 10 I will go into the process of personalising your nutrition, which involves investigating all these individual factors, tracking your food choices and the impact they have on your overall sense of wellbeing and symptoms.

But before we move into that next step, I want to talk about the other foundational lifestyle factors that may be muddying the waters and keeping us from seeing what is really going on with our health. Let's look at sleep, stress reduction, and exercise and movement.

CHAPTER 9

CLEARING THE MUDDY WATERS - LIFESTYLE FACTORS

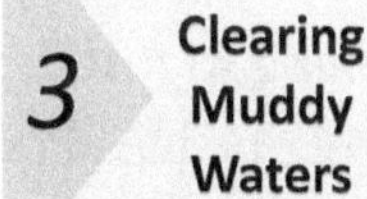

In health and in life, everything matters. You can eat the healthiest diet on the planet but if you are not sleeping well, if you are stressed, not moving enough you won't achieve optimal health. And taking it a step further: your relationships, being in nature, experiencing joy, having a purpose, finances, your career, your spiritual connection to something larger than yourself all contribute to your wellbeing. In this chapter I will take you through powerful lifestyle changes that, stacked on top of the healthy diet principles outlined in chapter 9, will make a big difference to your health and wellbeing.

Stacking with lifestyle factors

Sleep

Being able to sleep well is such a gift. To fall asleep effortlessly the moment you hit your pillow, sleep soundly through the night, and to wake up feeling fresh and well rested is a feat not many of us are able to achieve these days. Rather than waking up feeling fresh and well rested, for most people the alarm is literally a dreaded wake-up call which forces them out of bed, feeling groggy and already longing for evening so that they can find their way back into their warm, cosy bed. Although the morning fog lifts eventually, along with the desire to get back into bed, there are several reasons why it is important to make sure you optimise your sleep.

Sleep is the time where your body goes through growth and repair processes. These processes are essential for optimal neurological performance, memory performance, athletic performance, immune system functioning, musculoskeletal growth and repair, thyroid function, insulin resistance, cellular regeneration, stress resilience and more. Continuous sleep deprivation or lack of good quality deep sleep is harmful to the mind and the body by affecting all these functions negatively, paving the way for many serious health issues to arise. Heart disease, diabetes, hypertension, even cancer have been linked to long-term sleep deprivation.

It is estimated that 2/3rds of adults have some kind

of problem with sleep. Some of it is self-induced by choosing to do something else like working or staying up late, but often the lack of sleep is a result of underlying imbalances and/or poor sleep hygiene. Sleep hygiene refers to a set of practices that set you up for a restful night's sleep. Here are some recommendations for building better habits that lead to a restful and restorative night sleep.

Your circadian rhythm

As explained in the Powering Up step, your circadian rhythm governs your sleep and wake cycle. In addition to exposing yourself to morning sunlight, there are a number of other things you can do to keep your body clocks well-regulated and synchronised.

Waking up

- Use a dawn simulator alarm clock, which has lights that gradually brighten to avoid a jarring wake-up call.
- Don't hit the snooze button. Sleeping for those extra few minutes does nothing but provide you with fragmented sleep, which can affect your productivity later on in the day.
- Think some happy thoughts before you step out of bed. Be grateful for another wonderful day and all the goodness it will bring.
- Expose yourself to some bright light. If it is still dark out, use bright artificial light.

- Get physical. Walk the dog, do some yoga, dance a little.

Daytime routine

- Head outdoors at some stage during your day to get exposed to natural bright sunlight.
- Exercise regularly. It has been shown that regular exercise over a longer period of time results in better quality sleep – more on this later!
- If you must nap, do so in the early part of the afternoon rather than closer to evening.
- Keep regular mealtimes with an early dinner.
- Dim the lights when it gets dark outside. This is your body's cue to start winding down. Exposure to bright lights after this will upset your internal clock by tricking it into thinking it is daytime.
- Wind down after dinner and avoid activities that are highly stimulating or work related.
- Avoid screens (computers, tablets, smartphones, TVs) at least one hour before bedtime. These screens emit blue light that disrupts your melatonin production. Melatonin is the sleep hormone that rises at night, getting you ready for bed. Grab a (relaxing) book instead!
- Install F Lux (www.justgetflux.com), which is an app that automatically adjusts the blue light as well as your screen brightness in the evenings.

Bedtime routine

- Keep regular sleep timings. Turn in at about the same time every night (preferably around 10:00 – 10:30) and get up at about the same time every morning.
- Individual sleep requirements are very personal but most people require a minimum of seven to eight hours a night. Remember that most of our deep sleep occurs early on in the night, so going to sleep well before midnight is best.
- Keep your bedroom cool and as quiet and dark as possible. Blackout curtains are best.
- Reduce your exposure to Electro Magnetic Frequencies by turning off the Wi-Fi, your phone, computer, devices, and TV plug in your bedroom.
- Practise some breathing exercises before you go to sleep to activate your relaxation response:
    - Breathe deeply through the nose for five minutes, inhaling to the count of three and exhaling to the count of six.
    - Practice left nostril breathing for a few minutes by placing the index and middle finger of your right hand on the space in between your eyebrows and closing the right nostril with your thumb. This activates the parasympathetic nervous system which helps you to relax and calm down.

Your diet

- Eat a real, wholesome food diet as described previously and appropriate for your individual requirements to make sure you provide your body with the right fuel. This is a foundation for good health overall, which covers the ability to sleep well.
- Avoid caffeine or anything else with caffeine in it post lunch. Caffeine is metabolised in different people in different ways but drinking it in the latter part of the day can disrupt your ability to sleep.
- Avoid alcohol after 4 p.m. It has been shown that even the moderate consumption of alcohol as long as six hours before bedtime can affect wakefulness during the second half of sleep.
- Have a high protein bedtime snack around half an hour before bedtime to maintain stable blood sugar levels if blood sugar fluctuations are a problem for you.

As with most things in life it takes commitment and effort to achieve the results you are looking for. Sleep is a result of good health but also a requirement for maintaining it. I highly recommend making it a priority so that you can start reaping the wonderful benefits of experiencing good night sleep on an on-going basis.

Exercise

Our bodies are designed to move. If we look at our ancestors, they had a daily routine that ensured they were getting all the exercise they needed. They walked, sometimes ran, lifted things, squatted down, got up and manoeuvred their way through natural landscapes. They did not have to make a special effort to move their bodies.

In contrast, we tend to sit around most of the time. We sit behind our desks, in cars, on sofas or chairs. Our daily movement is often pretty much limited to walking from our home to the car, from the car to our office or store, and so on. Which is why we need to make a special effort to move our bodies through what is known as **exercise**: *an activity requiring physical effort, carried out especially to sustain or improve health and fitness.*

I am a big fan of an ancestral approach towards exercising. This approach looks at the way human bodies have moved for millions of years because that is really how we are genetically programmed to move even today. In a nutshell, this includes the following components:

- Move regularly at low to moderate intensity: around 2 to 5 hours a week of walking, cycling, swimming at around 55 to 75% of your maximum heart rate. What this means in practice is around 30 minutes a day. This could be as simple as walking 15 minutes into one direction and then walk back every morning or evening and you're done.
- Short sessions of functional movements, a few times a week for up to 30 minutes. Functional movements are

exercises such as lunges, push-ups, squats, pull-ups, and sit-ups.

- High intensity interval sessions, going all out once a week for about 10 to 12 minutes. Research has shown that occasional short bursts of all-out effort have much more impact on fitness (and even weight loss) than longer lasting, medium paced jogging, for example. This can be done through a set of sprints, on a bike, cross trainer or even in a pool.

As you can see, exercising according to these principles does not mean spending hours in the gym or hours walking or jogging. My suggestion is to try different things. Sign up for a yoga class, commit to a daily early morning walk when the air is crisp and the world around still moves a bit slower. Put on your favourite song and dance or jump on a rebounder. Or try Tai Chi, salsa lessons, tennis, kickboxing, or pole dancing. The possibilities are endless. And if jogging is your thing, so be it. Everyone is different and at the end of the day it is about figuring out what works for you.

Why do you exercise? – A study in motivation

We all know how important it is to exercise. And just as a reminder, these are some of the benefits: exercise improves brain function, it lifts your mood and reduces depression, it boosts confidence, helps with sleep, stress, energy, immune function, it balances neurotransmitters, and it has a beneficial impact on the gut microbiomes. Yet, despite all these benefits, it can be hard to stay motivated to exercise.

In a study on exercise and motivation participants were asked why they exercised. While 75% gave answers such as "to feel healthy", "to live longer", 25% said they exercised because of how it made them feel: they responded with answers such as "to feel grounded", "energised" or "centred". The interesting thing in this study was that the first group actually exercised 32% less than those participants that had made a connection between exercise and immediate benefits such as more energy and feeling more positive. By recognising the connection between exercise and immediate benefits, exercise moves from being a chore to a gift: something you engage in willingly because of the way it makes you feel.

One of my clients had a particularly difficult time finding the time and motivation to exercise. She had been an athlete as a teenager and well into her 20s and 30s but her demanding career, gradual increase in weight, and subsequent knee issues made it difficult for her to find joy in exercising. Until she tried a yoga class. The slow-paced private class guided by a yoga teacher had her feeling calm, more balanced, and stable in her body. Exercise was no longer a chore; it became something she looked forward to because of the immediate and noticeable benefits that she experienced.

I can very much relate as yoga has been my choice of

exercise for many years. As I moved into a different stage of life, however, I started gravitating (probably because my body needed it) to more cardiovascular exercise and weight training. And I experienced the immediate benefits of doing a combination of HIIT and weight training in a group setting. While yoga has me feeling calm and centred, my HIIT sessions make me feel energised. You can see how it is personal and dependent on your life's circumstances. You too can find your perfect form of exercise simply by experimenting and letting your body guide you to what is appropriate for you at a given point in time.

Movement

While exercise is an activity you choose to do for a certain period to enhance health and fitness, movement is the non-exercise activities that you engage in throughout your day. Considering that our lives are relatively sedentary compared to our ancestors, it helps to consciously implement some strategies to increase movement. Here are some creative and fun ways to do so:

- **Practice "active" sitting**
  When sitting down to work, be mindful not to slouch or lean back against the back of your chair. Just the act of sitting up straight, without back support helps to engage the core muscles. Sit at the edge of your chair with your spine straight, your

shoulders squared and your feet firmly planted on the floor. There are special tools that allow you to move while sitting such as an "active chair", an inflatable balancing disk, or sitting on an exercise ball instead of a chair. Some fitness experts advocate balancing a book on your head while sitting so that you actively lengthen and expand against gravity.

- **Set an alarm**

  By putting an alarm on your phone or computer every 20 – 30 minutes you will be reminded to get up and move your body. Aim to move from sitting to standing at least 32 times a day as a guideline.

- **Find a variety of movements**

  Make a list of easy to do sets of movement that you can frequently and consistently practise for a few minutes during the day. A few burpees, jumping jacks, jumping on a rebounder, short walks, stretching, shaking it out, lifting dumbbells, etc. are all great options. Get creative and remember this is meant to be non-intense movement for short periods of time only. When it comes to movement you want to favour **frequency and consistency** over duration: it is better to walk one mile three times a day vs walking three miles once a day.

- **Invest in a standing desk**

  To avoid sitting at your desk for long periods of time you can invest in a standing desk. These have become an increasingly popular tool to increase the health benefits associated with standing vs sitting. Some people take it a step further and use a treadmill desk that allows you to walk while working, which may be a bit far-fetched for most of us. Creating your own standing desk by using a crate or something similar to increase the height of your computer or work surface can work just as well and is a great way to get started.

- **Wear a pedometer or step tracker**
  Research has shown that wearing a pedometer, like a Fitbit, Oura Ring or using the step tracker on your phone improves the amount of walking you do in a day. The act of keeping track and measuring something helps to increase performance.

Stress reduction

Stress comes in many forms and has a profound effect on all the different systems of our body. We tend to think of stress as it is caused by **external factors** such as work deadlines, relationship problems, getting caught in a traffic jam or financial worries. There are, of course, many other sources of stress that are internally or externally driven, like chronic inflammation, infections, toxic burdens. Finding these stressors is part of a personalised health optimisation approach and will be further covered in chapter 11. For now, let's talk about learning how to effectively manage the more mental/emotional external stressors and how to reduce the effect they have on our lives.

There are two ways of dealing with elevated stress

levels: one is to reduce the underlying cause, which is often easier said than done. The other way is to implement techniques that can help you to better manage the stress in your life. The Mindfulness Morning Routine that is outlined in chapter 8 is one of the best ways to set you up for a more stable and stress-free day. Additionally, here are a few more of my favourite tools:

- **Get organised**

  It can be very helpful to set up a routine for activities such as getting up, eating, exercising, and sleeping. Organise yourself in such a way that you can stick with this routine every day.

  I highly recommend using a to-do list to stay organised and on track without last minute pressure. Every morning, write down what you need to get done that day. Start with a few easy things to get going and then tackle the more important items. Check off your tasks as you complete them and whatever you are not able to finish, move it over to the next day.

- **Switch off**

  With modern technology and gadgets, we are continuously connected. This can be a good thing but from a stress management point of view it makes sense to set some strong boundaries with respect to your email and phone. Set your email account to check for new messages only a few times a day so that you are not continuously alerted whenever a new message comes in.

Use your weekends to switch off from work completely and refrain from checking your mails or social media.

Similarly, you can choose to follow what Tim Ferris, in his book *The 4-Hour Workweek* calls a "low information diet". It is so easy to get caught up in negativity and stressful news as soon as you switch on the TV or open up a newspaper. This in itself can add to stress levels and it can be helpful to be selective about what you read or watch. I personally choose not to read the newspaper to avoid starting my day with negativity.

- **Breathe**
We rarely pay attention to the act of breathing. It just happens, naturally and without any effort. The beautiful thing is that you can consciously slow down your breath and activate your parasympathetic nervous system, which is the "rest and digest" part of your nervous system. Some basic deep, abdominal breathing with an emphasis on lengthening the out-breath does wonders for your body and mind. Try to spend 5 to 10 minutes breathing deeply every day to balance your nervous system.

Relaxing Breathing Exercise:

This breathing exercise helps to relax the body and the nervous system. Whenever you feel tense, upset, a need to relax or just before bedtime practise this technique to clear and calm your mind.

Sit upright with your back straight and your hands placed in your lap, palms facing up. Place the tip of your tongue softly against the back of your upper front teeth where they meet the gum ridge. Relax your body, close your eyes and begin by exhaling fully through your nose. Inhale deeply through your nose to the count of 4, hold your breath to the count of 7 and exhale completely through the nose to the count of 8.

Repeat this cycle about 5 times and then return your breath to normal while you continue to sit for a few moments with relaxed awareness of the sensations in your body.

- **Get a massage**

  Massages are relaxing and here is why: they stimulate the vagus nerve (the long cranial nerve that runs from your brain to your belly), which activates the parasympathetic nervous system, thereby lowering cortisol levels and raising oxytocin, the "love" hormone. Who doesn't need some of that good old "loving feeling!" A massage once a week to once a month should give you tremendous benefits.

- **Journal**

  A journal is a private space where you can record your thoughts, your innermost feelings and your dreams. I have maintained a journal for a few years now and although I don't write in it every day, on days that something is troubling me it helps me tremendously to gain clarity. Some of my most important insights and a-ha moments have come through the simple act of writing out my thoughts. As I write, anxiety and feelings of being overwhelmed just melt away and I am able to retrieve my focus and put things in perspective. I consider it to be an important part of my self-care routine.

I recognise that putting in place these lifestyle factors is not always an easy thing to do. Many of my clients are high performing individuals with extremely busy, stressful jobs and little time outside their work to look after themselves. Part of my job is to make them understand that life gets so much easier when these elements are put into place. That somehow, because of enhanced self-care and the resulting boost in energy, focus and productivity, time seems to free up more. It is a worthwhile investment to make for an easier, more balanced life that can positively impact other areas such as career, finances, and relationships.

Remember, you don't need to have this all out sorted today itself. You can pick one of these pieces and focus on that one first. Perhaps start with being more mindful about your food. Then stack that with another piece, like exercising regularly. After some time, when new habits have seamlessly been integrated into your normal routine, add something else and so on, until one day you look at your life and realise all the changes you have made and how they have positively impacted your life.

CHAPTER 10

GET PERSONAL

4 Making It Personal

Beyond the basics

You're eating a clean and wholesome, nutrient-dense diet, you are supporting good quality sleep, you are moving your body, and you are consciously working on lowering your stress levels. After just a couple of weeks of such wonderful selfcare you are likely to experience tremendous benefits. Chances are your digestion has improved, mysterious aches and pains have gone away, your energy is more stable, and you are feeling good physically and mentally. For many people, doing this clean-up is all they needed to do to get back to feeling great. If so, keep at it. You have found a balanced way of eating and living that supports your health and by just experiencing the benefits you are going to want to continue on this path.

For other people the beneficial impact is there, and very noticeable, but certain symptoms remain. David, who we met in Chapter 8, had initiated most of the principles I outlined above on his own for a while now, and he felt so much better than he did when he started. He was feeling lighter, sleeping better, but certain symptoms remained: he continued to feel stiffness in his knees, still had occasional episodes of palpitations, and his digestion continued to trouble him.

After doing a full functional assessment, looking at David's family history, his own health history, his current diet, and other factors, it was clear that the area we needed to zoom in on were his gut and the microbes that lived there. David had several clues in his health history that indicated his gut and microbiome health had been compromised: frequent antibiotics and other medications, periods of high stress, IBS type symptoms, and his family history showed digestive issues as well. I helped him to further personalise his diet approach to support gut healing with a short 30-day gut reset protocol that eliminated additional gut-irritants such as grains and legumes.

To gain additional insights into what was going on "under the hood" David did a functional GI test that assesses digestive function, gut inflammation, and imbalances in the gut microbiome. When this test came back it was immediately clear that David had a compromised gut barrier, an overgrowth of certain potentially pathogenic bacteria and reduced amounts of beneficial bacteria.

These findings correlated with his digestive symptoms and signs of inflammation and allowed us to get very targeted with his nutrition and supplement regime. We brought in gut healing supplements that help to heal the gut barrier and support the immune system, targeted probiotics and prebiotics to encourage the growth of beneficial bacteria. Slowly and gradually David began to experience consistent and normal bowel movements, the stiffness in his knees disappeared, he stopped having palpitations, and he finally felt he was in a good place with his health.

If, after implementing to the best of your ability the foundational diet and lifestyle principles you are still experiencing nagging health issues or you would like to take it to the next level in terms of optimising your health, it is time to move to the next step: personalising your approach. Like David, many of my clients need to go through a period of certain tailormade dietary changes to allow healing to occur, to restore nutrient deficiencies, support their "weak links" or to rebalance their gut and microbiome.

To determine the appropriate nutrition and lifestyle recommendations for you, we need to get to know you. **Truly** get to know you. And for that we need to gather as much information as we can. Here are the things we need to consider before crafting a set of recommendations uniquely tailored for you.

The information gathering process

What's your "poison"

Almost everyone can name certain foods that just don't agree with them. You may not understand why, but eating these foods brings up uncomfortable symptoms like allergic reactions, acidity, bloating or a headache and you try to avoid them as much as possible. Here are some examples:

- Caffeine: it makes you feel like you're bouncing off the walls. You love drinking coffee, but it leaves you jittery and feeling hyper. On those occasions that you have coffee in the late afternoon, you have a difficult time falling asleep at night.
- Prawns: the last time you ate prawns your face swelled up and you got itchy all over.
- Alcohol: even the slightest bit of alcohol gives you a headache.
- Beans: don't even go there. The severe bloating that follows is just not worth it.
- Spicy foods: they give you indigestion and acid reflux.
- Sweet foods: these trigger heart palpitations.
- Fried foods: you just can't manage to digest these well and you feel uncomfortably full and even nauseous after eating them.

These are all examples of foods that you would naturally

avoid, for obvious reasons. They are also important clues into what may be going on "under the hood".

The three broad categories of food reactions are food allergies, food sensitivities, and food intolerances. The first two categories are immune mediated and involve a set of reactions that kick in shortly after eating the trigger food. In the case of a true allergy this immune reaction can be severe and even life threatening; for example, in the case of a peanut allergy. A sensitivity also involves an immune reaction but symptoms may be less severe and food sensitivities can often be resolved through an elimination diet and simultaneous gut healing and immune system support.

A food intolerance does not involve the immune system and is mostly the result of genetics, a compromised digestive function, or imbalances in the gut microbiome. Food intolerance symptoms tend to take a bit longer to appear. An example of this is lactose intolerance in people that lack the enzyme to digest lactose or stomach pain or bloating after eating certain foods.

Symptoms, especially when triggered by your diet, are important clues as to what may be going on internally that is causing these foods to "disagree" with you and therefore what needs to be addressed. Taking note of trigger foods and their respective symptoms as described above is a first step in uncovering underlying imbalances.

Using one of the above examples to illustrate this:

beans are known to cause gas in most people. They contain certain types of carbohydrates that feed gut bacteria that use these carbohydrates to generate gasses. This is a normal process but in people who have an overgrowth of bacteria in the small intestine (the upper part of your digestive tract), this bacterial fermentation process happens too high up in the digestive system, where gas has no chance to escape the normal route and causes highly uncomfortable bloating. One client described it as feeling six months pregnant and needing to unbutton her pants to accommodate that sudden waistline expansion after meals. In that client's case, a simple review of symptoms along with the triggers made it clear that small intestinal bacterial overgrowth (a condition also known as SIBO) was likely to be her issue. We confirmed this with a SIBO breath test and took the necessary steps to address the bacterial overgrowth and the reasons for it.

Maintaining a food journal and taking note of symptoms as and when they appear may help you to make connections. If it is confusing, enlist the help of a functional nutrition practitioner who is trained at identifying connections, spotting problem foods or food categories, and crafting personalised therapeutic healing diets.

Your health history

Having a detailed look at someone's health history is essential in a personalised wellness approach and unfortunately, this important step is still not used to its fullest potential in many holistic wellness practices. I can't begin to tell you how many times a client (or I) had an a-ha moment when talking through their life story: connecting the start of their symptoms with a certain life event, or finally understanding why their health issue was just not getting better.

One of my clients was diagnosed by a naturopathic doctor with SIBO. The doctor in question had done great work in identifying the symptoms, getting the right tests done to find the reason for his digestive distress, and prescribing the right medication as well as nutrition recommendations. Only his symptoms kept coming back. When I did a full review of his history and took time to discuss with him his lifestyle, his diet habits, and his hobbies the likely reason for the recurring symptoms became quite clear. He was a businessman but also a passionate bodybuilder. To support this rigorous training routine and body composition he ate 6–7 large meals a day and took a variety of supplements. All of this had been wreaking havoc on his gut. There was simply no rest time for his digestive system to clear out food (and bacteria) between meals and he was in desperate need of gut repair. He needed help in marrying the required nutrition changes with his bodybuilding goals and finding cleaner alternatives to his bodybuilding supplements. He needed a much more personalised approach than just a diet sheet and medication. And as soon as he learnt to navigate all this his digestion started to improve and the bacterial overgrowth cleared up permanently.

In a health history review we look at everything that contributed to you being who you are today: your family history, the health of your parents at conception, the health of your mom during pregnancy, your birth, your diet as a baby, a child, a teenager, your past health issues, surgeries, your life events, your environment – we try to capture as much information as possible in order to get a full and comprehensive picture of you. There are so many things hidden within your life story that help uncover what your weak links and imbalances at this point may be and where we need to look to address these imbalances.

Blood chemistry test data

Most people, especially those with health issues or health conditions, have done lab tests. These tests, if they are less than six months old, can throw up some important clues as well. Even if a certain lab marker is within the standard lab range and therefore considered to be "normal" from a conventional perspective, when looked at through a functional lens it can show potential imbalances. Most standard lab ranges only flag pathological issues. A functional lab range looks at the results from a perspective of optimal vs suboptimal. If lab tests are not available, I often request a standard blood test as part of the initial review for this reason.

Food journal

Part of the assessment involves a few days of carefully tracking food and your symptoms that are happening daily. Food journaling is the simple act of mapping out what you eat or drink throughout the day along with the symptoms that you are experiencing and when. Symptoms such as energy fluctuations, congestion, throat irritation, a nagging cough, bloating, pain, itching, hives, or headaches, when reviewed alongside a food journal, can provide powerful insights.

This diet journaling step has helped me to pinpoint blood sugar imbalances or clients' intolerances to certain food compounds such as oxalates, histamine, or fermentable carbohydrates. It can also highlight nutritional imbalances and the potential for improvements.

The matrix

The matrix is a tool that is used in Functional Medicine and Nutrition by practitioners to map out what my mentor, Andrea Nakayama, a leading functional medicine nutritionist and educator in the U.S.A., so aptly calls: the person's story, the soup, and the skills. Information from your timeline, your symptoms, lab tests, and food journal are all used to complete the matrix.

The first part of the matrix includes all the factors that set the stage for your current health situation, such as family history, life events, prior health issues or illnesses.

It also covers the triggering events, which are the events or circumstances that triggered the onset or worsening of your existing health condition or symptoms. And it has the mediators, which are the factors that either make you feel better or worse.

The second part of the matrix is the "soup" section, which is like a brainstorming tool. Physical and mental symptoms, diet patterns, lab markers, clinical insights, and anything else which is relevant and based on the detailed health assessment is entered in this section under the main areas of fundamental biochemical imbalances. Together it forms an interconnected map that highlights the main areas of imbalance and where to focus attention to begin restoring balance.

The third part of the matrix is the "skills" section: it outlines the main diet and lifestyle areas and is used to note down what is lacking in these areas and what can be done to help.

Together, the information on this one-page document becomes a tool that helps a functional nutrition and lifestyle practitioner to connect the dots and identify key areas of focus. It informs the next steps of the personalised health optimisation process and becomes a quick guide to turn to when the health optimisation process is met with challenges, or to simply add more relevant information that becomes available during the implementation and tracking process.

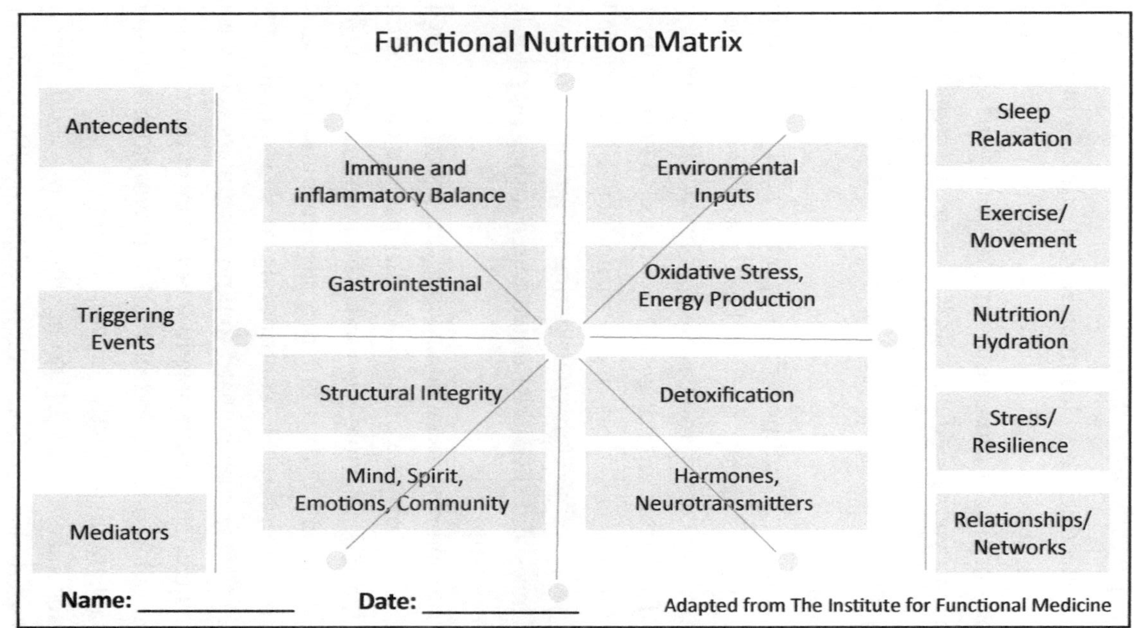

The sections of a Functional Nutrition Matrix (designed by Andrea Nakayama of the Functional Nutrition Alliance).

Your personal reset

After collecting and documenting all this information and doing a thorough review of the main imbalances and potential root causes it is time to tailor your diet and lifestyle to your specific needs. Here are the steps:

Step 1

Elimination

In chapter 9 I outlined the importance of eliminating certain foods that are fuelling health issues. Those foods included processed foods, sugar, refined vegetable seed oils – foods that are not good for anyone to have in their diet. Gluten and dairy were mentioned there as well as they are very often contributing to gut and immune imbalances and should be tested to see if they play a role in your symptoms.

Based on the detailed assessment process outlined above, there may be other foods that require elimination for a period. It could be foods that you are obviously allergic or sensitive to but may also include foods that you are not aware are contributing to your imbalances. Some of these may be hard to pinpoint unless you work with a qualified health practitioner and even then, it may take an additional period of food and symptom tracking to establish what exactly the culprits are.

After many years of doing this work, I can often tell, based on symptoms alone, what specific foods or compounds are contributing. For example, if a client has a history of kidney stones and one of his or her main complaints is joint pain, I would ask them to eliminate foods that are high in oxalates. If there is a history of diabetes in the family, signs of blood sugar swings and high fasting blood sugar on their lab results, a blood sugar balancing diet approach is warranted. This usually means adjusting carbohydrate intake and implementing blood balancing practices such as including healthy fat, fibre, and protein with all meals and snacks.

If digestives issues like severe bloating and acid reflux or IBS are the main complaints, especially after eating foods that contain fermentable carbohydrates (FODMAPS, which are foods such as beans, legumes, dairy, onions, garlic, mushrooms, apples or mango), I may recommend removing foods that are high in these FODMAPs. If someone has an autoimmune condition, a short-term elimination healing diet that excludes foods that impact the gut barrier and the immune system, such as grains, legumes, nightshade vegetables, and nuts and seeds may be warranted. Histamine intolerance is a very common root cause for symptoms such as hives, itching, a racing heartbeat, and nasal congestion after eating. Removing high histamine foods while working on underlying root causes is necessary to deal with this type of food intolerance.

In many cases and especially when gut issues are involved or correlations are not yet very clear, I recommend

30 days of a plant-powered paleo way of eating. This means removing gluten, dairy, grains, legumes, alcohol, and caffeine. A plant powered paleo way of eating includes plenty of vegetables, some fruits, nuts and seeds, animal protein and healthy fats and naturally removes all potential gut irritants, helps to balance blood sugar, calms the immune system, and boosts nutrient density. Yes, it may be one of the popular "diets" out there (and we are not a fan of dieting), but I have had a lot of success with incorporating this as a 30-day reset with many of my clients, and there are a lot of resources available in the form of cookbooks, recipes and even meal delivery services.

After a 30-day elimination reset individual foods are reintroduced to identify symptom triggers (see step 6).

Step 2

Boosting nutrient density

After looking at eliminating foods that are triggering or contributing to your symptoms, the next step is to boost the nutrient density of your diet to ensure you are getting all you need from the food you eat. Some of the top nutrient dense foods in terms of vitamins and minerals are foods that no longer have a prominent place in our diet, like organ meats or small fish. Other nutrient dense foods are green leafy vegetables, shellfish, meat, and eggs, so if you tolerate these, it pays to include them in your diet regularly. Plant foods contain many plant-specific nutrients, such as polyphenols and fibres that have many health benefits and that help support a balanced and diverse gut microbiome.

Eating a varied diet is key. Different types of vegetables, protein, and other foods have different nutrient profiles and the more diverse your diet, the more vitamins, minerals, and plant-based nutrients you will get into your body. If you are a creature of comfort, you may try to step out of that comfort zone and experiment with different vegetables, fruits, nuts, or seeds.

Step 3
Supplements

In an ideal situation we obtain all our nutrients from the food we eat but in reality there often is a mismatch between our genetic requirements and our dietary habits, lifestyle and environmental factors. High levels of stress, existing health conditions, toxic exposure, frequent travel, inflammatory imbalances or a lifelong diet of refined foods, caffeine or alcohol can all contribute to a higher demand for certain nutrients. A compromised digestion can interfere with your ability to absorb nutrients, imbalances in your gut microbiome can impact nutrient status and genetic mutations can cause an increased demand for certain cofactors.

You are genetically adapted to get your nutrition through food. There is an obvious difference between the synergistic effect of nutrients as they exist in whole foods and taking isolated nutrients in supplement form. Your first and foremost goal should therefore be to reduce the nutritional gap as much as possible by striving to eat the best possible diet and the highest quality of nutrient dense food alongside managing lifestyle factors, and optimizing your digestion and microbiome health.

Once you have built a strong foundation in these areas you can examine your bio-individual need for added support. A standard lab test can throw up some useful information and functional testing (see the next chapter) can help identify an additional need for targeted supplements that help support immune function, hormone balance, digestive health, gut barrier healing or detoxification- and antioxidant support.

Step 4

Gut Barrier Healing

This support can come in the form of gut healing foods like bone broth or supplements and special herbs. Choosing these additional gut supporting factors is again a personalised process.

Step 5

Lifestyle practices

In the previous chapter we looked at the importance of incorporating good lifestyle habits in the area of exercise, sleep, and stress management. Despite your best efforts you may not be at an optimal level in one or all of these areas. In this personalisation step it may, therefore, be necessary to work on these factors in greater detail. This could mean incorporating personalised breathing practices, working with a physiotherapist to address structural issues, a therapist to deal with past trauma, or a career coach to address work related stress.

Step 6

Tuning in, tracking and reintroductions

One of the key parts of a personalised health optimisation process is the ability to tune in, track, and adjust where needed. As you are making changes to your diet and lifestyle, you want to record how you feel and track the impact these changes are making on your symptoms. You can easily do this on your own with the help of a food and lifestyle journal or you can enlist the help of a functional nutrition and lifestyle practitioner that can make connections that you may be missing.

Especially when food triggers your symptoms, as is the case in many digestive related issues or immune reactions, journaling these symptoms can help to provide important clues and further insights. This feedback then forms the basis for tweaks and fine-tuning to further personalise the approach.

After the short (usually 30 days) elimination and depending on your progress you may be able to start reintroducing foods back into your diet. At that stage tracking your symptoms is important to see which foods continue to be triggers and which foods are okay for you to include back into your diet. A systematic reintroduction process of individual foods will help you to isolate foods that continue to trigger symptoms and need to be eliminated for a longer period or even permanently in some cases.

CHAPTER 11

ROOT CAUSE TESTING

5 Testing

Up to this point you have been using diet and lifestyle modifications and perhaps targeted supplementation to support your personal health building journey. Diet and lifestyle adjustments are extremely powerful and, in many cases, they are enough to turn around your health, boost your energy, productivity and focus, and resolve nagging health issues. A lot of this work can be done by you, sometimes with the guidance of a functional healthcare professional who is able to see the connections, can identify underlying imbalances, and structure a more targeted dietary and supplement strategy.

Sometimes, when there is a lot "in the mix" and more data is required or when symptoms remain even after a targeted diet and lifestyle approach, it can be necessary to do a deeper investigation into the nature of underlying imbalances. This is the point where functional testing comes in. Functional tests are tests that are not diagnostic in nature; they are not used to find a disease. They are used to identify root causes: imbalances that drive the disease process and contribute to symptoms and that are not immediately obvious just by looking at a standard blood test or symptom evaluation.

Every symptom in your body is driven by underlying imbalances. Sometimes the connections seem far-fetched but they are there. To use a few examples: anxiety can be triggered by gut imbalances, cardiovascular disease can be linked to microbiome disruptions, Alzheimer's disease is a multifactorial condition that has its roots in many different imbalances.

At some point in my own health journey, in 2013 I was at that exact point where I knew I needed to dig deeper. I had embraced a gut healing, nutrient dense, anti-inflammatory diet, was on top of my exercise, stress management, and sleep, yet I was still struggling with lingering digestive issues, like bloating, changes in bowel movements, and low energy levels. I had completed a health coaching training and was looking for more education to sink my teeth into. When I came across Functional Diagnostics Nutrition I knew this was what I needed: a practitioner training programme that teaches you how to use functional testing to get to the root cause of health issues. During the training programme you use yourself as a test case and so I ran a few tests on myself under the guidance of a mentor.

One of these tests was a detailed GI test and the other one an adrenal hormone panel. The adrenal hormone panel showed that I was dealing with HPA axis dysfunction, which is often the outcome of long-term exposure to chronic stressors, and which explained the fatigue that I was dealing with. The GI test revealed the nature of this chronic stress: I still had signs of a leaky gut, and bacterial and parasite infections in my digestive tract. The best diet on the planet (which I pretty much was eating at the time), was not able to negate the impact of these infections. They had to be treated. I chose to go the herbal route and did a six-week herbal protocol to kill the unwanted bacteria and parasites and break down the biofilm that these microbes build around themselves for protection. I simultaneously brought in gut healing supplements to restore the intestinal barrier and encourage the growth of important beneficial bacteria.

All the while I continued with my nutrient dense, gut healing diet. It got a bit worse before it got better but I slowly began to feel like me again. My stomach flattened, my sleep deepened, my energy became more consistent, and my digestion normalised. A repeat test a few months later showed a much better picture of my gut function and microbiome – I finally had managed to clear what had been at the root of my problems for a long time.

Functional, root cause testing is a powerful way to

identify root cause imbalances in the areas such as hormones, detoxification, gut imbalances, nutrient deficiencies, and metabolic processes. There is, however, a reason that it is one of the last steps in a personalised health optimisation journey. Often, doing the foundational nutrition and lifestyle work outlined in the previous chapters is enough, especially if you work with an experienced practitioner who is able to identify imbalances based on a thorough intake and symptom review.

If you do come to a point, like me, where you hit a roadblock, it may be time to work with your practitioner on testing. There are many great tests available, and the choice of testing depends on your needs. As with everything else, it's personal! To give you an idea of the types of functional tests that are available and how they can be of use, here are some examples:

1. Blood chemistry analysis

A standard comprehensive blood test, looked at through a functional lens, can help reveal underlying imbalances such as inflammatory processes, impaired detoxification, nutrient deficiencies, hormonal imbalances, or digestive issues. A comprehensive blood test should include a comprehensive blood count (CBC) with white blood count differentials, markers for liver and kidney health, a detailed cholesterol panel with homocysteine, thyroid markers, inflammatory markers such as CRP, an iron panel, and basic nutrients such as vitamin D, magnesium, folate, and B12. I work with many clients in Europe and other parts of the world where conventional doctors don't want to do such extensive testing because of insurance guidelines. However, there are labs that are offering comprehensive health checkups outside insurance at a reasonable cost. It makes sense to periodically use this option to get an overview of where you are.

2. GI and microbiome test

A functional GI test analysis uses a stool sample to find signs of impaired digestive function, gut inflammation, intestinal barrier dysfunction as well as imbalances in the gut microbiome. It can identify the presence of pathogenic micro-organisms, but also general imbalances in the gut microbiome, such as an overgrowth of potentially pathogenic bacteria and a lack of beneficial ones. There are a few options in the market for doing these tests. Choosing the right one depends on your goals and a good practitioner will know how to choose one that is evidence based. There are a growing number of gut microbiome tests that offer direct to consumer analysis of the entire bacterial population within your gut microbiome and based on your results, offer recommendations to help boost diversity or the growth of beneficial bacteria with targeted diet strategies. As of the time of writing this, there is still a lot we don't know about the gut microbiome and results have to be interpreted accordingly. These tests can offer helpful insights but if you are struggling with your digestion, you may want to choose a test that includes markers of digestive function and that also looks for the presence of parasites, yeast or viruses.

3. Food sensitivity test

A high-quality food sensitivity test can help identify your level of reactivity or sensitivity to specific foods. It is this heightened reactivity that can fuel inflammation and cause digestive, skin, neurological, joint, and other symptoms. A note of caution: I have seen many clients who have done food intolerance tests on their own and have received back a laundry list of foods that they had a sensitivity to and were told to avoid. These clients were often overwhelmed and having a difficult time removing all these foods from their diet. Having a long list of food sensitivities is actually a symptom that points at a compromised gut barrier, which has the immune system working on overdrive. Rather than trying to figure out how to navigate a diet that excludes so many foods, using a personalised elimination reset diet (see chapter 10) and working on restoring gut barrier integrity usually does the job of calming down the immune system and reducing food intolerances.

4. Organic acids test

This test analyses urinary organic acids: a class of compounds that are formed during metabolic processes in the body.

Increased or reduced levels of these different organic acids can help to identify a need for certain nutrients, bacterial imbalances, yeast or fungal overgrowth, mold toxicity, oxidative stress, or the presence of other toxins in the body. It is a great screening tool to help pinpoint problem areas. Organic acid tests have helped me to correlate client symptoms with the presence of yeast overgrowth, heavy metal toxicity, mold, and a genetically driven tendency to build up oxalates in the body.

5. DUTCH (Dried Urine Test for Comprehensive Hormones)

The DUTCH test provides a very comprehensive overview of sex and adrenal hormones and their metabolites, melatonin, and a few organic acids. It is an extremely useful test to get insights into hormonal imbalances, including HPA axis dysregulation, and identify targeted ways to support hormonal balance through nutrition, supplement, and lifestyle interventions.

6. Nutrigenetic test

A good quality DNA test identifies unique DNA sequences in some of your genes that have been studied in detail and that are linked to an individual's risk for developing certain chronic disease or altered metabolic processes. These results can then be used to recommend diet and lifestyle changes that have significant evidence for being able to impact the disease risk.

7. HTMA (Hair Tissue Mineral Analysis)

The HTMA test uses a hair sample and provides insight on mineral and toxic metal levels in the body and how well the body can currently excrete toxic metals. It is a great health screening test for a variety of health issues impacted by mineral imbalances and toxic heavy metal burden.

The above is just a sample of tests available that can help to further personalise your health strategy and allow for a more targeted approach. Choosing the right test depends on all the information gathered thus far: your full functional assessment, your symptoms and your goals and the impact of a reset or elimination diet. It is an important next step in the root cause investigative process. Additionally, certain tests, like a Nutrigenetic test, can also be very informative and insightful for someone who is feeling good and has no obvious health complaints. Such a test can help identify potential "weak links" and provide information on how to support yourself going forward in the best way possible.

Similarly, you can now get insights into your aging process. Tests like TruAge show you what your biological or epigenetic age is (as compared to your chronological age, which is determined by the number of years you have lived). By having insight into the speed with which you are aging you can incorporate changes to slow down this process and by repeating the test, see the impact your diet and lifestyle changes have on your biological age.

Testing as a preventative measure, or to help sustain good health and high performance into the future is part of what I like to call the "tinkering" process, and this is the subject of the next chapter.

CHAPTER 12

SUSTAINING HIGH PERFORMANCE

6 **Tinkering**

Your perfect routine

When done right, the entire personalised process outlined above is going to provide you clarity on what you need to do to feel your best and sustain that for the rest of your life. Restoring imbalances can take some time, especially when these imbalances have formed over a long period of time but by putting in place the right diet and lifestyle factors that are based on your unique needs, you will eventually wake up one morning, step out of bed and realise: I feel great. At that point there will be three elements to your health routine that will help you to continue to feel that way.

1. Your non-negotiables

By now you know what makes you feel good and what

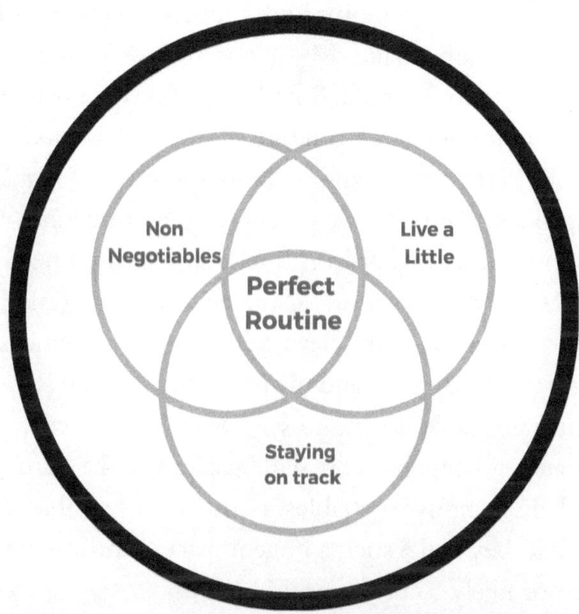

doesn't. You will know the things that you need to have in place to be your optimal best. These are your "non-negotiables" – the things you don't want to mess with, or at least not too often. It could be eight hours of sleep a night, your mindful morning routine, a jog in the park five days a week. You may need weight bearing exercises to support bone health. Or avoid sugar or gluten, limiting alcohol to once a week or maybe not at all. When allergy season comes along you will have to take extra care to support your immune system by way of targeted supplements.

In my case, I don't tolerate dairy well, but I can have the occasional piece of goat cheese. Too much gluten triggers digestive symptoms and I function best on a low to moderate carb intake. My gut is my weak link and I always need to look after it. Some of the keystone beneficial bacteria in my gut microbiome are at lower levels and I need to include certain foods and prebiotics in my diet regularly to help boost them. I have certain genetic mutations that predispose me to higher iron levels, an increased need for folate, B vitamins, vitamin A, magnesium, and omega 3. I need to make sure my diet meets these requirements. I don't do well with stress and my Mindful Morning Routine is a non-negotiable for me to stay mentally balanced.

Whatever happens, you will need to make sure you uphold these non-negotiables as much as possible. And given that they make such a huge impact on how you feel, this is not likely to be an issue.

2. Live a little

Let's face it: life happens and there will be times when you throw all caution to the wind to splurge, indulge or "cheat". On a day-to-day basis you should have in place carefully curated nutrition and lifestyle practices that help you to stay well. These nutrition and lifestyle practices are based on your unique requirements, your genetics strengths and weaknesses, environmental influences, and your health history. Once you have all these bio-individual practices firmly in place, you will be able to step out and enjoy an occasional treat, let go while on vacation or spend a decadent weekend with friends in Italy and still feel healthy.

Remember, it is not what you do once in a while. It is what you do every day that matters. So, having a glass of wine on the weekend, indulging in a piece of cake on your birthday or going all out on your holiday is likely to be okay. It may have to be a gluten free piece of cake if you are gluten intolerant: if eating a certain food is going to make you feel uncomfortable for days, it is a different question. In that case that food will be in your non-negotiable list and is best avoided all the time.

3. Staying on track

If staying on track is challenging and the occasional indulgence becomes a regular one, it may be time to tap back into your motivating factor. In chapter 6 I talked about creating a foundation by digging deep and finding your unique Why for embarking on a personal health building journey. Keeping this why, your goals and your intentions close by and visible will help remind you why you want to live your optimal life, to be radiant, fit, and energetic and live with purpose and joy. Knowing why this is a priority will make it easier to make the right choices for yourself.

You can't manage what you don't measure

Part of staying healthy and picking up on important cues that indicate the need for course correction is to measure what is going on in your body. Waiting for the signals to appear is usually not a good strategy because symptoms arise when underlying imbalances are well underway. And therefore, you want to periodically check in and keep an eye on where you are at.

What to measure depends on your prior issues, your "weak" links and what you know you need to stay on top of. If you are prone to blood sugar issues you may want to measure blood glucose levels. If your gut is your weak link, a periodic gut and microbiome assessment could be helpful. Here are some of the tools and devices that you can consider:

1. A periodic full blood chemistry analysis, viewed through a functional lens.
2. The symptom questionnaire at the end of this book to see what's lingering and what needs more support.
3. A Continuous Glucose Monitor to assess blood sugar balance as well as bio-individual responses to food.
4. A gut microbiome analysis to monitor the impact of your diet and lifestyle on the diversity and composition of your microbiome.
5. An assessment of the different areas in your life and where you need more focus. Examples are physical activity, career, finances, relationships, access to nature, spirituality, social life, creativity, etc.
6. Sleep tracking devices such as the OURA ring or Whoop band to measure key markers such as heart rate variability, sleep patterns, and daily activity.

Tinkering

Another word for tinkering could be biohacking, which is a term that has become popular in the last couple of years. Tinkering (or biohacking) refers to fully tapping into your potential with health and longevity hacks. Some like to call it the do-it-yourself biology for human enhancement. This can be as simple as using diet and lifestyle interventions, like intermittent fasting or taking a certain supplement that has been shown to slow down aging. There are many great tools and interventions that can help you make further improvements to your health. I consider this stage to be the icing on the cake and a truly fun way to experiment with some of the latest health boosting tricks to see how it can further enhance your health and wellbeing.

At the time of writing this book there is a lot of focus on anti-aging. People are tinkering with supplements and practices that have shown to help enhance your health and your life span. And I am all for that, as long as you have the foundations that are outlined in this book in place. I can't stress enough how you need "fertile soil" for seeds to achieve their optimal potential. And it is the same with specialised supplements or other health hacks: for these practices or interventions to have the maximum impact you need a strong foundation in the form of a healthy, balanced body. And let's not forget that having a healthy, balanced body is one of the most effective anti-aging treatments!

With that foundation firmly in place, let's look at some of the things that you can experiment with to further enhance your health and slow down your biological clock:

1. Sound therapy

Sound is energy and specific sound frequencies can activate certain mental states and balance the nervous system. An example of this is the use of Brainwave audio sessions to shift the brain into a specific state and as such induce enhanced focus, relaxation or sleep. Other sound or music therapy types include gong baths, the use of singing bowls, drums, tuning forks, and the human voice.

2. Touch therapy

I mentioned earlier the power of having a massage: not only does it boost circulation and detoxification, it helps to shift you into a parasympathetic rest and digest and healing state. In a similar fashion, there are devices that you can strap onto your wrist or ankle, like the Apollo Neuro or Neurosonic, which provides silent vibrations that soothe the nervous system and help you recover from stress.

3. Heat therapy

Sauna bathing involves exposing yourself to high heat in an enclosed space. The resulting increase in body temperature triggers a range of cellular responses that have well researched benefits on circulation, detoxification, cardiovascular health, immune function, and brain health.

4. Light therapy

Exposing your body to infrared and near-infrared light can result in enhanced skin health, recovery, immune support, and overall healing. It has been shown to be beneficial in exercise recovery, skin improvement, and the optimisation of sleep.

5. Cold therapy

Like with heat, exposing your body to cold temperatures triggers a range of physiological mechanisms, also referred to as the cold shock response. Benefits include reduced inflammation, improved metabolic health, improved mood and cognition and beneficial changes in the gut microbiome.

6. Sleep therapy

Sleep plays such an important role in health and wellbeing, as discussed in chapter 10, and there are many tools and devices that can help further enhance the quality of your sleep. Some examples are special mattress covers that lower the temperature of your sleep surface, grounding mats, or blue light blocking glasses that minimise your exposure to blue light after sunset.

7. Breath therapy

Breath therapy is the use of specific breathing techniques to induce healing states and balance within the body, mind, and spirit. The ancient science of yoga includes a wide range of different breathing techniques and there are many other forms of breathwork therapy that can help support general well-being.

8. Removing environmental stressors

Electromagnetic frequency radiation is continuously being emitted around us by our electronic devices, appliances, electrical wiring, and power lines. As technology advances, levels will continue to increase. There are several companies that have created devices to help mitigate the effects of electromagnetic radiation. Products range from little stick-ons that you can stick to your phone or laptop or larger devices that you can place in your home.

9. Aromatherapy

Essential oils are compounds that have been extracted from plants and can be used therapeutically. Inhaling aromas from these essential oils, or using them topically can activate the limbic system, which is the area in your brain that is the centre for memory and emotions. Different essential oils induce different states of being that can range from feeling energised and uplifted to peaceful and grounded.

10. Sublime emotions

Finally, let's not underestimate the power of simple happiness hacks such as experiencing awe, joy, bliss, or true love. No investment required!

To experience these sublime emotions, you really don't have to travel far. All it takes is walking around with awareness and looking at the world with fresh eyes, noticing things such as the beauty of a tall tree, the vibrant colours of flowers on your dining table, a piece of art or the sun streaming through your window, the smell of a cup of freshly brewed coffee. It's about cultivating the same sense of presence and awareness that is generated by the Mindful Morning Routine. If you make it a habit to periodically stop, take a breath, and notice the environment around you, you will be able to find pleasure in the little things and call in joy on command.

Try to follow your passion. I described how over the years I pursued the things that made me feel excited and alive, that got my heart rate up. It eventually birthed an entire new career and allowed me to turn my passion into work. You can make a conscious effort to do more of the things that you love; take a course, or join a club or community where you can learn more or engage in your hobby.

And last but not least: cultivating love. Feeling true love, THE highest and purest force of life, is the ultimate happiness hack. Consciously tapping into a feeling of deep love and appreciation for the people in your life, a pet, and most of all: yourself. Ultimately that is the most powerful part of living your most optimal life.

Final Words

At the risk of sounding like a broken record, I am going

to repeat what I consider to be a crucial aspect of anyone's health and happiness journey: everything matters. We are wired to get excited at the thought of shortcuts and exciting new modalities but these work best when stacked on top of the basic fundamentals.

Doing the basic work is not sexy, I get it. Some may even consider it boring. Using aromatherapy or infrared light, or supplements is way more exciting than eliminating foods. Please flip that switch in your head. Take it from me and my many years of experience that the basic work is essential and that it can become exciting, especially once you notice the dramatic impact it has on your health.

Healthy food can be delicious. Experiment, make it your mission in life to make healthy food taste good. I have seen many a naysayer, including my own children, get excited at the sight of a big rainbow coloured salad as long as it was accompanied by their favourite dressing and perhaps a piece of grass-fed steak. One of my clients was lucky to have a wife who loved cooking and the pictures he sent me of his meals used to make me drool. Needless to say, his 30-day elimination reset was easy for him.

If you need support, look for a functional, integrative or holistic minded healthcare practitioner. If they ignore the fundamentals, keep looking. Even if they are excellent functional doctors, if they move straight to testing without digging into the diet and lifestyle habits, they are missing an important point. I have seen many clients who have worked with great functional doctors but without building that diet and lifestyle foundation and getting the necessary support with implementation and tracking, they did not get the results they were looking for.

A great healthcare practitioner knows when to refer out. Whether it is to a health coach for support with day-to-day implementation of diet and lifestyle changes, a specialist to work with on specific health conditions or a nutritionist who can work with therapeutic diets. Or maybe a meditation teacher, a holistic dentist, physiotherapist, hypnotherapist, chiropractor, or psychologist.

The healthcare clinic of the future is one where all of this is found under one roof. But even in the absence of such a holistic health centre, you can create a team of practitioners around you. Make sure that your main practitioner is part of such a referral network.

And finally, remind yourself periodically, why this is all important. Revisit the vision you created for yourself and remember that looking after your health is a critical part of achieving this vision as well as your highest potential. By doing this, you can change your life and the lives of the people around you and be part of an important ripple effect that truly has the potential to change the world.

Be well!

ABOUT THE AUTHOR

About 15 years ago Monique embarked on a personal health-building journey that led her to dive deep into the world of functional health and nutrition. With an MSc degree in Personalised Nutrition, certifications in Functional Nutrition, yoga and health coaching, as well as trainings with some of the world's leading Functional Health Practitioners, Monique has been able to develop a deep understanding of functional nutrition, bio-individuality, and how to take an evidence-informed, holistic and root cause approach to addressing a wide variety of health concerns.

Monique works virtually with clients across the globe and her approach involves creating highly personalised diet, lifestyle and supplementation strategies to restore homeostasis, the use of high-end functional testing to identify core imbalances, and providing on-going support to fine-tune and ensure compliance and success. Monique's area of passion and expertise is the use and interpretation of GI and microbiome tests and restoring gut and microbiome health as a core component of all health building programmes.

Originally from the Netherlands, she currently lives in India with her husband but has spent the last 28 years as an expat living in eight different countries across the globe.

She is a proud mom of two college-going children and toy poodle, Nacho. When Monique is not buried in health research studies, books, or podcasts, you can find her in the kitchen, outdoors or catching up with family and friends over a good meal.

SYMPTOM QUESTIONNAIRE

Rate each of the following symptoms based upon your typical health profile for the past 30 days.

Point Scale:
0 = Never
1 = Rarely, Effect not severe
2 = Occasionally, Effect not severe
3 = Occasionally, Effect severe
4 = Frequently, Effect not severe
5 = Frequently, Effect severe

SYMPTOM QUESTIONNAIRE

Head

Headaches		Faintness	
Dizziness			
		Total	

Nose

Stuffy nose		Sinus problems	
Hay fever		Sneezing attacks	
Excessive mucus formation		Loss sense of smell	
		Total	

Nails

Spoon shaped		Brittle, cracking	
Discolored		White spots	
Lines/Stripes			
		Total	

SYMPTOM QUESTIONNAIRE

Hair

Hair thinning		Hair loss	
Loss of outer eyebrow hair		Premature greying	
Easy hair pluckability			
		Total	

Skin

Acne		Hives, rashes	
Dry skin		Bumps on back of arms	
Flushing		Excessive sweating	
		Total	

Immune

Colds		Flu	
Chronic infections			
		Total	

SYMPTOM QUESTIONNAIRE

Genitourinary			
Frequent or urgent urination		Brittle, cracking	
Discharge		White spots	
		Total	

Eyes			
Watery/itchy eyes		Yellowing eyes	
Swollen, reddened, sticky eyelids		Bags, dark circles	
Night vision problems		Blurred vision	
Loss peripheral vision			
		Total	

Mouth/Throat			
Chronic coughing		Gagging frequently, throat clearing	
Sore throat		Hoarseness	

SYMPTOM QUESTIONNAIRE

Mouth/Throat			
Swollen/discoloured tongue		Burning tongue	
Coating on tongue		Chewing problems	
Canker Sores		Fever blisters	
Cracks corner of mouth			
		Total	

Heart			
Irregular/skipped beats		Rapid/pounding beats	
Chest Pain			
		Total	

Lungs			
Chest congestion		Asthma or bronchitis	
Shortness of breath		Difficulty breathing	
		Total	

SYMPTOM QUESTIONNAIRE

Energy/Sleep			
Fatigue		Lethargy	
Hyperactivity		Insomnia	
Sleep disruptions			
		Total	

Neurological			
Poor memory		Confusion	
Poor concentration/"brain fog"		Poor physical coordination	
Loss of balance		Tingling in hands or feet	
Stuttering or stammering		Slurred speech	
		Total	

SYMPTOM QUESTIONNAIRE

Ears

Itchy Ears		Ear aches, ear infections	
Drainage from ear		Ringing	
Hearing loss			
		Total	

Digestive Tract/Gastrointestinal (GI)

Nausea		Vomiting	
Diarrhoea		Constipation	
Alternating diarrhoea & constipation		Bloating	
Belching		Gas/flatulence	
Heartburn		Upper GI pain	
Lower abdominal pain			
		Total	

SYMPTOM QUESTIONNAIRE

Joints/Muscle/Bone			
Pain or aches in joints		Arthritis	
Stiffness/limited movement		Pain or aches in muscles	
Feeling of weakness or loss of strength		Restless legs	
Bone pain		Broken bones	
		Total	

Weight			
Underweight		Overweight	
Obese		Weight loss (>5-10 lbs)	
Weight gain (>5-10 lbs)		Fluid retention	
		Total	

Emotions			
Mood swings		Anxiety, worry, fear, nervousness	
Anger, irritability, agitation		Premature greying	
		Total	

Key: the higher the score, the greater the impact on the individual.
- 0-15 Fair
- 16-25 Moderate
- 26-50 Major
- >50 Severe